HEALERS
unlimited

Magnetic Energy
Healing of the Future

FRONT COVER

Colin's guide, Dr Wilbur Sargesson steps in to assist with the healing of a patient.
Dr Sargesson was Danish and passed back into Spirit in 1879.
(Note the blur of the hands due to the incredible speed at which they are moving).

Colin R Lambert

HEALERS
unlimited

Magnetic Energy
Healing of the Future

Colin R Lambert

April 2000
Peaceful Living Publications
PO Box 300 Tauranga
NEW ZEALAND

First Printed - March 2000

ISBN 0-908807-04X

National Library of New Zealand cataloguing-in-Publication data
Lambert, Colin, 1920
Healers Unlimited: Magnetic Healing
Natural Healing
Alternative Medicine
Alternative Healing

Peaceful Living Publications
P.O.Box 300
Tauranga
New Zealand

Printed in Tauranga, New Zealand by KALE PRINT.

Contents

Preface

As I pick up my pen to write these first few words as a preface to this, my fifth book, I ponder upon what may be found on its pages by the time I sit down to pen the last chapter. There have been many times during the writing of my other books, when, after sitting at my desk watching the pen flow across the paper for quite sometime, I have sat back and said to myself, "It must be about time I checked back to see what has been written."

On some of those occasions I have been quite surprised to discover certain phrases and ideas which appeared to be quite new to me, and I would think, "Did I really write that?"

Much of the time of course, I am consciously recording in the written word some of the wonderful experiences I have had the pleasure and privilege of being part of during my twenty trips out of Auckland's Airport, or the equally exciting times spent conducting public lectures and teaching classes from one end of New Zealand to the other. Since my previous work "You Too Can Heal" was first published in June 1993 for instance, I have held similar meetings in several parts of Australia, in Hawaii, England, Canada, and at two separate times in U.S.

But at other times the pen flows effortlessly across the page and I am well aware that something is being written which is not necessarily a normal part of my thinking pattern, and I know that there is one who is impressing upon me certain thoughts and understandings which he wishes to be given to the people of planet Earth in order to help to lift it out of the quagmire of mistrust and degradation which its people have brought it down to.

Judging by the incredible number of phone calls and letters I have received from readers of "You Too Can Heal" and the way in which they have described their reaction to those words, it would seem that the success of this method of bringing truth to those who are ready to accept it has been far beyond anything I would have expected.

It is my intention to include on the pages of this work, some extracts from a few of those communications to allow you to share with me some of the joy which has filled my being as I have read them or listened to them on the phone. The word inspire, or its derivatives, is a word which crops up frequently, and I have long since lost count of the number of times I have heard someone say something like, "Mr Lambert, your book has inspired me to go out and learn to be a channel for the healing energy so that I can bring new health and hope and upliftment to those in need."

Sometimes it is a simple "You have been an inspiration to me" But whatever form it comes in, it is still a very humbling experience, and I know that once again it has been proven to me that the time and energy spent in holding a pen above a sheet of paper and watching the ink sprawl its way across the page has been more worthwhile than I could ever have hoped for.

My one prayer at this time as the marathon effort of writing yet another book begins, is that the words which will fill it will once again "Inspire" someone out there to make the sort of changes in their life which will bring about for Mother Earth what is commonly referred to as the great New Age of Light and Enlightenment.

Colin R Lambert
New Zealand
1999

Father of Medicine

From the writings of Hippocrates, the Father of Medicine
460 - 357 BC

It is believed by experienced Doctors
that the heat which oozes out of the hand, on being applied to the sick,
is highly salutary ...
It has often appeared while I have been thus soothing my patients,

**AS IF THERE WERE A SINGULAR PROPERTY IN MY HANDS
TO PULL AND DRAW AWAY FROM THE AFFECTED PARTS, ACHES
AND DIVERSE IMPURITIES,**

by laying my hand upon the place, and by extending my fingers towards it.

Thus it is known to some of the learned
that health may be implanted in the sick by certain gestures,
and by contact,
as some diseases may be communicated from one to another.

This is what we now term

'MAGNETIC HEALING'

1. GIVE IT A NAME

Wherever I travel either within my home country or overseas I am always bombarded with a multitude of questions about my work as a healer and a teacher, and so it is my desire at this time to write a book which will answer many of those questions before they have even been asked. There is one which I have not yet heard of course but feel sure that many will ask me when they see the title of this book "Healers Unlimited".

So perhaps this would be a good place to begin, for if I answer it now at this early stage, then that will be one question less you will need to ask me if I happen to be in your area at some future time and have the pleasure of meeting you.

And yes, before I do, let me just say that if you are wondering whether that will ever happen then I can only say that depends on you more than it depends on me. You see almost everywhere I have been on this wonderful planet I have travelled there simply because some searching soul in that area has written or phoned me to ask if I would come to their area to lecture and to teach them and their friends the art of Magnetic Healing. On more than one occasion however, I have travelled overseas to a particular area simply because I have been asked either by telephone or letter if I would give someone "Absent Healing".

Because of the result of that healing, the very happy recipient has sent me return airline tickets to travel to his or her home to be their guest. For those of you who may be reading this and do not understand the meaning of "Absent Healing" I will go into that subject in some detail in a later chapter.

But back to the naming of this book. While I have been doing what I call Magnetic Healing for about thirty years, I did not begin to show others how to do this work until 1987. Indeed, I was not really aware that it would be possible to do so, and it was not until I was asked to go to Maui to lecture at a dinner at a hotel and then try to show others how to do this work that I really gave any serious thought to this possibility. I must admit that after holding several workshops with around twenty students in each, I was even more surprised by the results than the students were. With a good "Guinea-pig" patient on the couch one of the students would be called up beside me, and having already found a negative area in the auric field of the patient I would say to the student, "You see where my hands are over this patient. I will take them away now, and I want you to place yours there and tell me if you feel anything different in that area".

The first time I did this I had no idea whether any of them would notice anything at all, leave alone come up against pressure between their hands in the same way that I had been doing on many patients over the past years. Imagine my surprise when one after another their hands would begin to shake and many of them would complain that they were having difficulty in bringing their hands together, while others would say, Its too heavy, I cannot lift it.

Sometimes I would have to take hold of their wrists and help them to lift the unwanted dross away from the patient, I soon came to realise that what I had taught myself to do was not something which was inherent within me alone, but was a natural ability within each of us just waiting to be recognised and tapped into.

Since that time I have lost count of how many such groups of students have sat in my class and one by one approached the patient, in most cases, not really expecting anything to happen. But time and again it has brought me great satisfaction, and very often, much amusement to just watch their reaction to the discovery that there really is a resistance to the movement of their hands as they approach the area of the body where there is some malfunction.

It was not long before I found myself saying to the group, "Look at that, Healers Unlimited, just waiting to recognise their inherent ability to be used as channels for the healing energy". So now you have it. Having watched many hundreds of students reacting to the pressure of the negative energy as they approach it, and having heard myself repeat these words to so many groups in several countries, I feel that I could not find a better name for a book which sets out to describe to its readers the simplicity of discovering for yourself this very simple yet effective method of bringing health, hope and upliftment to those in need. Hence the name, "Healers Unlimited".

You may well be wondering why, if putting out your hands to heal an ailing body is as simple as I have just shown it to be, there are not more people doing it, and why it is not recognised by the orthodox medical fraternity as a practicable method of treating their patients. There are many reasons why this is so, and much of this book will be devoted to answering those questions. Many times in my lectures and workshops my students would have heard me say, "you are exactly what you believe you are, and nothing more and nothing less than exactly that".

I would like to ask you at this time to sit back and give a little thought to that statement because I believe it is one of the most important observations I will be recording here. Take a good look at your own life. How did you come to be what you are? What sort of environment were you brought up in? Were your parents religious, and if so, what effect has this had on your life? Did they have an open mind on the possibility of there being an alternative to the normally accepted method of caring for the sick, or did they consider that visiting a doctor and being given a prescription for some particular drug or medicine of some kind was the only path worth following? And what about some of those people you know who belong to a different race. Why do their standards, their beliefs appear to be so different to yours? Did you automatically follow the beliefs and understandings of your parents, and did those of another race do the same, or have you used your time on Planet Earth in this particular incarnation to go to the trouble to think things out for yourself? The answers to those questions will tell you exactly why you are what you are. One thing I have learned in my nearly eighty years in this body, is the fact that the great majority of people are just too lazy to bother about what God gave them to think with. They find it much easier to accept what professor so and so said, or perhaps a statement from their Priest or minister, and all too many are even naive enough to accept a decree from their member of Parliament as being the whole truth and nothing but the truth. We tend to say, they are the experts, they must know.

But perhaps an even more important thing I have learned, is the fact that truth is the most unlikely thing you will be given by any of these people. I have come to realise that both science and religion know full well that once you discover truth they will lose you. Proving this statement will also become a substantial portion of this work. "The truth will set you free" is an old but very good saying. One might say that this in itself is truth.

Looking back at my own life, I see a little boy being taken off to Sunday School each Sunday, sometimes even having the privilege of going to lunch at the home of our minister. Everything was prim and proper and we children were expected to be seen but rarely heard. My eldest brother was ten years older than me and I have never forgotten the Sunday morning when a group of us was standing on the footpath outside the church talking to the minister after the service. My brother was telling him about someone he had seen driving a car much too fast, and in doing so used an expression which was quite often used at that time. He explained to the minister how he had seen this car travelling "At a whale of a bat". Mind you, I have no idea how such a saying came about, but we were quite happy that everyone knew that it meant the car was travelling very fast.

I can still see the puzzled look on my brothers face when the minister turned on him and said, "Oh Ted, you should not say that, that is blasphemy". Would you believe my brother is now 90 years young, and I am sure both of us have spent the more than 70 years since we heard that statement trying to figure out just what could possibly be blasphemous in those words. I think they may have gone quite a long way towards making both of us start questioning as to whether this was the sort of environment we wished to remain in for the rest of our lives. Maybe it was part of the reason why both of us have stepped aside from it long ago.

What I could never understand at that time was why I was told that the day you are born you are a naughty sinner and you should be kneeling to Him and asking for forgiveness. Forgiveness? What for? I did not know then, and I still don't. It was not until many years later when I first heard of reincarnation that I began to realise what was lacking in my life and in the teachings I had been brought up with. In other words, in the environment in which I had been born into.

Of course, I was not aware then as I am now, that little if anything really is an accident. Looking back now, if I had not gone through those experiences, then I would not have had any idea what I was talking about concerning these things. But having been there and done that has given me a more balanced appreciation of the many paths which it is possible for a human being to follow in his endless quest for truth. Mind you, even now I still do not understand that statement about being a naughty sinner the day I am born. At least not from the point of view of people I spent much of my childhood with anyway. These were people who would not even listen to the possibility that there may be some truth in the theory of reincarnation. So I used to ask myself just how, if I only come here once and have never existed before, could I possibly have sinned the moment I arrived? Was it something to do with Eve eating a forbidden apple? Did that make me a sinner too? Is their God not a God of love? Could He be so spiteful as to decree that from that moment on every child born on Planet Earth would automatically be a sinner in His sight. Surely this could not be a God of love.

And why must they deny the reincarnating of the soul in a physical body more than once. Did they think that soul could learn all the many lessons to be learnt in just one short sojourn in the physical form as a soul incarnate as the Bible puts it, with all the rest of that souls existence being spent as a discarnate soul. Thirty or more years ago I was practising hypnosis and many times I took my subject back through several past lives spent on the planet, some of them several hundred years apart and others a few months to just a few years between incarnations. At that time I found that by putting one of my subjects into hypnosis some months after the first occasion, then taking them back to certain dates which they had spoken about the first time, they invariably came up with the same information which they had given me previously.

This was all recorded on tape so it was easy for me to check any discrepancies in their stories, but try as I would; I could never find one. There was no way that someone could describe to me who they were, the name of their husband, wife, children, or friend at that time, the town and country they were residing in and a thousand little details about their life, and then come up with exactly the same details several months or even years later during a second session. It became quite obvious that they had to be describing those experiences as they saw them in what is commonly called their Karmic record.

I think it was this experience which did more to change my thinking pattern than any other single happening in my life. I came to the conclusion that if I were not being told the truth by those who most people expect to hear it from, then I would have to make the effort to discover it for myself. Perhaps of all the phrases I had seen in the Bible during my church and Sunday school days, the one which now meant the most to me was that short statement, "Seek and thou shalt find". The intervening years since that time have proved the truth of that statement. I have found a great deal of truth in my quest, but even now, as I often say to groups of people I may be lecturing to in a public hall, or smaller bands of students I may be teaching to become magnetic healers, the most important truth I know is the fact that I still know almost nothing.

Never make the mistake of thinking that you already know all that you need to know, for when you do that you cease fulfilling the purpose for which you incarnated in the physical form on Mother Earth. And I say this to both the scientist and the follower of any particular religious faith. A sign on the wall of my healing room makes this simple statement, "MINDS ARE LIKE PARACHUTES, THEY ONLY FUNCTION WHEN THEY ARE OPEN".

How true I have found that statement to be during those thirty or more years I have spent seeking, as they might say in court, "The truth, the whole truth, and nothing but the truth". There will be many stories I will tell within the pages of this book, which will prove to you too the truth of that statement. The medical people in particular who have turned a blind eye to many of the wonderful healings I have had the pleasure and privilege of being the channel through which the Universal Energy, Love-force, God-force, or whatever you desire to label it with, flowed through to the patient in order to bring about the restoration of health, hope and upliftment to the particular patient concerned.

It has not been an easy path to follow, but it has certainly been a rewarding one. There were times when I would have as many as 450 appointments in my diary. This would amount to about two months work, and it would worry me a great deal when I would pick up the phone and a very sick person on the other end, sometimes crying in their desperation, was trying to make an appointment in the hope that I would be able to discover the source of their problem and lift it away from their ailing body. How does one say, "Sorry, I am booked up for two months"? No wonder the hours in a day were never long enough.

But nowadays, while I still help a few needy people in this way, most of my time and energy goes into showing others that as the title of my last book and also my one hour video tape says, "You Too Can Heal". To watch someone who has never felt the energy flow through them step up to the couch in a teaching workshop and to watch the expression on that ones face as he or she suddenly finds they can barely bring their hands together because of the resistance between them as they approach the negative energy in that part of a patients aura immediately above the affected part of the body, is the sort of thrill and reward for my work which I would find difficult to express in words.

One of those occasions I have a very good reason to recall. This particular student was one who had come along to the class, not so much with the idea of learning to become a healer, but rather with the intention of proving that the whole thing was a farce. Sceptics such as this one can be very difficult to convince, but the way the day worked out meant that it was not necessary for me to prove anything to him at all. He did that for himself. When he came up beside me I showed him where to place his hands several inches apart above the body of the ailing patient on the couch, I then told him to slowly bring his hands together and to see what he could feel there. I had of course, already checked out the patient, so I knew exactly where to tell him to place his hands where he would feel the most effect.

But even I was not prepared for what took place a few moments later. I soon realised that not only was he feeling the negative energy between his hands, but he was obviously finding great difficulty in bringing his hands together, such was the resistance to their movement. Then came an explosion of words from his lips as he suddenly lifted both hands up in front of him and swung his body around in order to be able to throw away whatever he had picked up well away from the patient. The startled look on his face told me all I needed to know. It was very obvious that he had not expected to feel anything, and was in quite a state of shock at what had happened.

I am often asked whether it is necessary for a student to have total faith in the healing process before it would be possible for him or her to be able to feel the negative energy and to remove it from the patients aura. There was a time early on in this work when the answer to that question would have been a very definite yes. But I have since been shown that one should never just automatically assume anything. In You Too Can Heal I told the story of the patient who came to my healing room with several different problems and stood beside my couch for a few moments before climbing on to it. As he stood there he assured me that as far as he was concerned this sort of thing was just a lot of b**** magic, and the only reason he was here was because his wife was tired of him being sick and kept on nagging at him to at least give it a try to see if it would work.

It became quite clear to me that he had decided to come, not with the idea of receiving any healing from this "magic", but only so that he would be able to go home and tell his wife that as he had expected, nothing had happened, and then perhaps she would stop nagging him. But it didn't work out like that for him either. He turned out to be one of those very sensitive patients who could not believe what he was feeling in his leg as my hand moved along above it in order to clear the blocked arteries which were giving him so much pain and so many sleepless nights. But after sleeping like a baby that night he became one of my most ardent followers, and sent many ailing patients to me for healing in the following years.

Perhaps I should have realised from this that the same sort of circumstances could apply for someone who comes into a workshop where the art of healing is being taught as one who comes into a healing room. Could it be that the soul within the body is at that time saying something like, "It is time this stubborn physical form of mine was taught a lesson. I am getting tired of him thinking he knows it all. It is time he woke up and realised there is much more to life than he imagines. He is never going to learn the lessons he came here to learn this way."

And so he is guided, even against his will, to be put in a position where that stubborn streak is given such a beating that he finally backs down and finds within himself, perhaps with much difficulty, a level of humility he had not previously been prepared to admit he possessed. It is not difficult to draw a parallel between the one who enters the healing room quite sure that nothing will happen, and the one who joins a group of people in a healing workshop equally as certain that the whole thing is just a way for someone to make money, even if there is only a donation box at the door.

So let us go back to our student with the expression of shock on his face and a torrent of words flowing from his lips. You may be wondering whether all this had any permanent effect on the beliefs, and indeed the life of this one. In answering that question for you, I could do no better than to quote from a letter I received from him several months later.

"Last night was our fifth fortnightly meeting. We meet between the hours of 7:30 and 10 pm and have four or five tables going flat out during that time. There are about twenty to twenty-five healers at each meeting, and the number of people who arrive for healing is increasing with each meeting. Two or three come along to learn the magnetic healing techniques and the group continues to grow without a great deal of effort. There are some really strong healers in the group and it is very exciting to see them develop from a sceptical beginning to a confident total believer.

It is also quite fascinating to watch people who have spent a great deal of time and money to be trained in Reiki, Aromatherapy, Reflexology and other healing techniques ignore their previous training and practise only Magnetic Healing. Just watching them develop is so exciting that I believe I now know one of the reasons why you enjoy teaching people the technique.

Operating from home, I find my healing appointments are growing continuously with the majority of people being referred to me from other satisfied patients. My enjoyment at being able to offer ease and comfort grows daily, and some of the successes have been mind blowing and more than outweigh any failures. I will always be grateful and thank you for turning a confirmed sceptic into a convert of Magnetic Healing."

If ever I needed a good reason for titling this book "Healers Unlimited" then surely the foregoing would have to be it. I might mention that a short time after the writer of that letter attended my workshop and discovered his exceptional ability to be a healer, he invited me to his home town where I held a public meeting and showed about fifty colour slides covering everything to do with energy including pyramids, Crop Circles, Psychic Surgery in the Philippines, Kirlian photography, and of course, Magnetic Healing, followed by a demonstration on a patient.

Strange to say there was not a large attendance at that meeting, but those who did attend must have been very busy the next morning telling their friends what they had missed because I had to stay another two days to conduct one three hour workshop in the morning and another in the afternoon on each of those days. I do not like to have more than about twenty students in each class, and it was amazing how they sorted themselves out with the result that I finished up teaching seventy seven very keen people the art of Magnetic Healing over those two days, with all of the classes ranging between eighteen and twenty one.

It was from this effort that the "Sceptic" who wrote me that wonderful letter was able to build on and keep the interest on the boil in the weeks and months that followed. This sort of response is typical of what I find is happening where ever I travel, whether it is in New Zealand or some other country overseas. An ever increasing number of people are finally beginning to question what they have been taught, and finding that teaching was not nearly as close to the truth as they had been led to believe.

Just two days ago I travelled about ninety miles to a small town where I had been asked to go to teach a group of people. There was only twelve in this group, but their enthusiasm made up for their lack of numbers. Some of them were already practising some form of healing such as Reiki, but others had nothing else going for them other than their desire to be able to heal their fellow beings in need.

And after all, this is all one needs. Readers of my previous book may remember that I mentioned there that in every class I hold, I tell my students that the most important statement I will make all day is one which I found myself saying one evening at the end of a meeting of like minded people about thirty years ago. At the end of that meeting I had demonstrated Magnetic Healing on a patient, and a man came up to me a few minutes after

I had finished and said he would love to be able to do healing like that. This was one of those occasions when a reply will suddenly issue from my lips before I have even had time to think about what I should say to him. The simple answer which came back to him said it all. "THAT WHICH YOU WILL ACHIEVE, WILL BE IN DIRECT PROPORTION TO THE DEPTH OF YOUR DESIRE TO SERVE". If you have not already seen this statement before, then I would like to suggest that you take a deep breath and go back and read it again. Just as it is the most important group of words I speak to my students, in the same way it could well be the most important I will write here also.

Let me briefly explain to you the reason why I consider it to be of such vital importance. To discover within yourself the ability to be able to reach out your hands over an ailing body and feel the Love-force energy flowing through you to that body in order to return the damaged cells back to their normal state to allow the patient to be at ease instead of diseased is one thing, but I can assure you that to have the courage to do this in public and to advertise the fact that you are a healer with all the ridicule that can bring from those who think they know better than to believe that this could possibly happen is a very different story.

Each time I hold a class for a new group I find that most of them come up to the body on the couch and place their hands on either side of the area where I have shown them there is negative energy, and they will find it has become quite difficult to bring their hands together due to the resistance created by that energy. From this moment on, it would then be possible for that one to run their hands slowly through the energy field of anyone who has any form of health problem whatsoever, and to find the source of that problem and work to remove it. I often tell them that the only thing I know of that is wrong with Magnetic Healing is the fact that it is much too simple. This becomes a problem because most highly educated scientific or medical people KNOW that it could not be possible to learn all one needs to know about how to achieve the ability to heal in a three hour session. What they don't know is the fact that each of us already has this ability laying dormant within us just waiting to be recognised and accepted by the body.

Many times I have checked up some weeks or months later to see how many of a particular group are still practising healing, and the saddest part of my work is to discover that there is one here and one there, and maybe with a bit of luck another over there who are still placing their hands above the sick and bringing new health and hope to them as the healing energy flows through to the patient. But then I remember that in the group which these ones were a part of, there were several others who I watched come up beside me and place their hands over the patient and suddenly become ecstatic as they felt the energy flow through them.

Where were they now? What had happened to them? There were a few who I could immediately see were what I sometimes refer to as a "Natural", and I had told them so. I would have been thinking to myself at that time, "This is great. Here is another one who is being used as a channel for the Love-force just as if she had been doing it all her life." But how could one who has discovered his or her latent ability to be a healer, and knowing full well that they are now quite capable of helping someone who is ill to become well just throw it away as if it was of no real value to them.

I will tell you how. It is really very simple. They may have been overwhelmed by their discovery of that ability, and some females break down in tears on my shoulder, such is the emotional feeling which fills them. But just as every bright sunny day is followed by the darkness of the night, so the exhilaration brought on by this discovery, can actually change to one of fear as they contemplate the possible repercussions of continuing to do this work.

Perhaps they have gone home to a husband or a partner and told them of their newfound ability and how wonderful it will be to now be able to help those in need. They may not be prepared for the response they receive from that husband or partner. It may never have occurred to her that as he had not been there and really had no idea of what she was talking about, he would blurt out something like, "You don't really think you can heal someone. Do you think you are a doctor or something just because you go out to see some nutty guy who tells you that you can heal people. Get real woman".

If that sounds a bit rough, well, I can tell you, I know several who have had an experience like that, and some of them even worse. Well this is where we go back to the words which I told you would be the most important statement I would be writing here. That which you will achieve will be in direct proportion to the depth or your desire to serve. The one I have just written about is already beginning to wonder just how her neighbours and her friends far and near will react when they hear she believes she can heal. Will they also think she has gone around the bend and is losing her sanity? Unfortunately some of them will. They will be the ones like her husband who are totally ignorant of their own inner capabilities, and are at a total loss to understand someone who has discovered theirs and have a desire to make use of them in service to their fellowman.

Some of you will no doubt have heard of a man by the name of Samuel Hahnemann who was the founder of the method of healing called Homeopathy, but perhaps you may not have seen this quote from his writings. “When we have to do with an art whose end is the saving of human life, any neglect to make ourselves masters of it becomes a crime”. I must say I agree with him 100%. To discover that you are able to help someone who is sick in some way, and then not bother to do anything about it surely is a crime.

Just last week I was faced with a very good example of this. Three people came to my healing room. There was a lady about forty five years old, a more elderly lady and an elderly man who was the patient. As they walked into my room I had the distinct impression that I should know the younger woman and felt that perhaps I had met her at one of my meetings at some time. However, as you can imagine, I meet hundreds of people wherever I go, so I thought that perhaps she was just a little like someone I had met and did not bother to question her in that regard. The patient climbed onto the couch and after working for a while to clear away unwanted dross from his blood, my hand began looking for any other negative energy within his Auric field.

As it approached the lower torso I found it would not go any further, and it felt as if there was an invisible wall in front of it. I remember thinking that almost anyone should be able to detect a resistance to the continued movement of the hand as strong as that one was, so I decided to ask the young woman to come up and place her hands over her friends body in the same place I had mine after I removed them. This she did, and just as I was about to tell her what she should do next and what she should expect to feel as I always do for anyone who is attempting to find the negative energy for the first time, her hands began to shake and it was obvious that she was already sensing the same resistance which I had felt, and was drawing it together in readiness to lift it away from the patient. I was amazed to see her working like a professional healer as she lifted the unwanted dross and returned her hands to gather up some more.

Very soon she said, “There doesn’t appear to be much resistance there now. I think it is clear”. As she drew her hands away, I placed mine there again and was quite surprised to find that as she had suggested, it was quite clear. I asked her where she learnt to heal like that and was a little taken aback when she reminded me that she had been to one of my workshops to learn the healing technique when I had visited her town for that purpose some years ago. No wonder I thought her face looked familiar, and I was pleased to know that she was still very capable of using what I had taught her but felt I must ask her what was to me the obvious question. Why did you bring your friend to me when you could have done this in your own home? Have you not been using that wonderful ability to heal which you obviously have?

After a moments silence she said a little sheepishly, "Well, not really?" Please, can someone tell me WHY? How could someone know that they could put out their hands to help their sick friend and then decide to commit, as Samuel Hahnemann put it, the crime of not making themselves master of it, and in fact not even using it at all. After the telling off I gave her I had the distinct impression that she had decided it was about time she changed all that and made good use of her abilities.

I trust she will now find that the depth of her desire to be of service to her fellow-beings has been strengthened a little, and it will be easier for her to face any ridicule which may be thrown at her by those who have not yet lifted themselves above the inhibiting belief that we are mere flesh and blood and quite incapable of being used as channels for the Universal Energy which is everywhere and is free for all to draw on once they have moved the barriers which hold them in eternal ignorance of their true Soul-self within and the incredible abilities which that recognition can bring with it.

2. JOYOUS SATISFACTION AND DEEP FRUSTRATION

You may well ask how anyone's life could be filled with two emotions so positively opposed to each other as those, which I have used as a heading for this chapter. I can only ask you to bear with me for the moment when I tell you that you will no longer be asking that question by the time you have finished reading it. Basically, the former of the two comes from the many wonderful reports I receive from several different quarters. They may arrive by telephone, by letter, or by word of mouth. They may consist of information concerning the result of a healing I have given to a patient, either directly, or by the method I briefly mentioned as absent healing. They can be from someone who has read one of my books and wants to tell me about the affect the books content has had on them, or they may be from one of my students who is ringing or writing to describe to me one or more healings which he has successfully carried out.

The letter from the ''sceptic" which has already been quoted from would fit into that last category, but whichever source they come from they all bring with them an exciting mixture of humbleness and joyous satisfaction. Humbleness in the recognition that one who for several years in the earlier part of his life spent his time down dirty dark coalmines hewing coal, followed by twenty five years running his own painting and decorating business could have suddenly discovered after he had been on the planet for almost half a century, the latent ability to heal his fellowman laying dormant within him. Joyous satisfaction that he did not selfishly hold this unto himself, but spent much time and energy writing about it in the hope that the information he gave to the people through the writing of four books would result in others realising that this recognition was available to all who would diligently seek it.

But perhaps the most rewarding of all are those stories I hear from the many students who pass on to me the results of the healing they have done. As I approach my eightieth year I am aware that I am every bit as human as everyone else, and I know that the time must come when I will be called back home. Home to what I sometimes refer to as the real world, the world of Spirit. When this does occur I look forward to being able to look back and see those who I have had the pleasure and great privilege of being able to guide onto the healing pathway, going about their work of taking pain and suffering from the physical bodies of their fellow-beings, and at the same time raising their conscious awareness, and in some cases, as we have seen with the sceptic, passing on to yet another the recognition of their true soul-self within, and their ability to be used as channels for the healing energy. As this process continues, and I see the "Hundredth Monkey" effect beginning to take place, joyous satisfaction does indeed fill my soul and my very being, and I offer a humble word of thanks.

The time is after 9 pm as I sit here watching my pen scrawl its way across the page. But suddenly, a few moments ago I was jerked back to reality by a noisy telephone beside me suddenly bursting forth into life. I picked it up and I just had to laugh when I heard what the man on the other end was saying to me. He began by telling me that he was ringing me from a very small town just out of Invercargill which is at the very bottom of the South Island of New Zealand and about one thousand miles from my home as the crow flies. Then he went on to tell me that he was just ringing to thank me for writing such wonderful books. He had read two of them but did not know that I had written two others or that I had a video tape which showed people how they could become Magnetic Healers. He immediately asked me for the price and my address so that he could send me a cheque for them. When he told me why he was ringing me, I said "Would you believe I am sitting here writing about people who ring me to tell me how much they have enjoyed reading one or other of my books". As I pointed out in my last book, nothing ever happens by accident in this work.

Just yesterday I received a letter from the other end of New Zealand near the top of the North Island, and perhaps it would be a good idea if I was to copy a portion of it to show you once again how more and more people are changing their thinking pattern and daring to look at new ideas which are often contrary to those which are recognised by orthodox science and religion.

"Dear Mr Lambert, I am proud to advise I was recently fortunate enough to be lent your very informative book "WHY" to read from a work colleague. Bravo and my congratulations to you for being free with sharing your experiences. I am particularly impressed with the fact that this was published some years ago, 1970 I think, when this would have been looked upon by most as untruthful. These days I think more and more people are finally realising we all have a body and a soul and our destiny is within. I also found "WHY" easy to read, and it is exciting to know more and more knowledge and information is becoming more readily available for us to learn about Spirituality.

I am thirty years old and over the last few years have been on my own Spiritual journey, but as I advise my friends, not in a religious sense. It has given me confidence to finally feel some inner peace within myself and it has allowed me to be in control more with my everyday decisions and destiny. The search for me has just begun in finding answers, and I am enjoying this journey for the first time in my life".

As I read that letter it occurred to me that as the writer had stated that she was just thirty years old, that meant she would have been born in 1969. In that year I sat at my desk and penned the words for my first book "WHY". Little could I have imagined that thirty years later I would be receiving a letter concerning the book from one who was in the process of entering the Earthplane once again in a tiny new body.

The foregoing letter arrived yesterday, but today the postie brought another, this time from a city in the South Island approximately 350 miles north of where this evening's phone originated. Once again we see that ever increasing desire to search for truth, and the recognition that it will not be found within the limiting dogma of a religious organisation, but deep within oneself where it lies waiting to be recognised and tapped into for the enlightenment of all. When the great Master Teacher we refer to as Jesus told the people that the Kingdom of God was within them, I am sure that was exactly what he meant. Why else would He say to those who accused Him of blasphemy by saying that He was God, "Ye are gods". The implications of these statements are profound, and a full recognition of their importance by the inhabitants of planet earth in general would be enough to bring about the wonderful New Age of light and enlightenment which has long been spoken of and sought by many.

But let us look at a portion of today's mail and see what the lady who wrote it has to say. "Dear Colin, I have just been reading your book "Here's Why", and I am very excited about it. 21 years have passed (1978) since you wrote that book. A lot must have happened since then. Did you write more books? Do you teach here in New Zealand? How can I help, and are you the one who will teach me, or will it come from within or both? Do you know if there is a group of like-minded people in my area?

I had to leave Holland fourteen years ago to come to New Zealand with my husband and four children. There was no room for expansion and growth in the sheltered family life where I came from. I am very thankful for all the people I met in New Zealand from all kinds of backgrounds, different beliefs and cultures. I learned so much and still it is only a little bit of the things I don't know. I do know that if I had all the knowledge of the world and did not have love, it would be of no use.

Currently I am a member of the Methodist Church and also a Theosophist. Sometimes I wonder why I am going to Church where they are so ignorant and feel secure to stay that way. Then I wonder if by sending light to the people in the church, if that is my job to help them in growing. I don't know. I will be so thankful if you have time to write back to me. May the love we are sharing spread its wings and fly across the earth and bring new joy to every soul on the planet. May the blessings of my Lord shine on every one, and may we all see the light within".

Wow ! So much wisdom in one small letter, yet at the same time a degree of confusion. Which path do I take? How do I get there? Will someone show me the way? If someone was to ask me why I spend endless hours of my life writing books and travelling all over New Zealand and several other countries around the world, the simple answer I would have to give them would be to tell them that I do it because I realise there are so many confused souls wherever I go who are diligently seeking answers to the questions which we find in the foregoing letter. If I can bring a little light into the lives of those seekers of truth, then that time and energy spent will have been well worth the effort.

About three months ago I drove my vehicle to Wellington which is at the bottom of our North Island, and took it with me on the car ferry across Cook Strait to the South Island. In the first town I went to I stayed in the home of a lady who had written to me some time previously for healing. I had worked on her several times during the following weeks, and while talking to her on the phone from my home, it had been arranged for her to organise a public meeting in a hall where I would show colour slides and then demonstrate Magnetic Healing on a patient, to be followed the next day by a workshop where I could show interested people how to become healers.

This lady had a daughter in her late teens living in another city further south, and she asked me if I could do what I could for her as apart from any physical problem she had, she was also in the grip of those soul destroying chemicals we call drugs. The weekend I visited her home coincided with a visit from her daughter, so I was able to speak to her and ask her if she would like to come along to a workshop to see if she was able to become a healer. I got the impression she thought something like that would be way out for someone who was living the only sort of life she knew, but as the students filed in for our first class, I was quite amazed to see her among them.

When the time came for her to come up beside me and put her hands out above the patient in the area I indicated to her, I was thrilled to see the expression on her face as her hands began to quiver and it became obvious she was having quite a problem trying to bring them together. After a little coaxing she managed to do this, and then with some effort, slowly lifted the dross from the patient's aura and threw it away.

I have seen this happen many times around the world wherever people have gathered to attempt to learn the technique of Magnetic Healing, but somehow I felt this was different. It had a very special feeling about it. Here was one who I felt was about to be lifted from the ground floor to the executive suite at the top. A move which had the potential to bring about an unbelievable change in her life. The firm planting of her feet on a new path, A whole new level of understanding. A giant step toward the recognition of her true soul-self within, and the realisation of the reason for her incarnation.

Since that time, her handyman father, at her request, has made her a folding aluminium healing couch which has been sent down to her so that she can carry on with the healing work which she now enjoys doing. The last time I spoke to her mother, she told me through tears of joy, that not only had her daughter given up the drugs, but was so well that she no longer needed the drugs which her doctor had been prescribing for her health. To add to this her father found himself having to make a second couch because mum is also doing healing in her home since my visit.

All of the above is of course, a part of that "Joyous Satisfaction" we find as a heading to this chapter. But what about the "Deep Frustration" which forms the other half of that heading? Surely all of this could have brought nothing with it but joy. So let me relate to you a story which is filled with both of these emotions. On the first day of February 1998 a Maori lady from Auckland, our largest NZ city and about ninety miles from my home, brought her eighteen-month-old daughter to me for healing. For the past nine months she had been having epileptic fits. Most days there would be as many as six or seven and several times she nearly lost the child as she would stop breathing temporarily. She informed me that her daughter was under the care of what is looked on as being the best children's hospital in the country, the near new Starship in Auckland. The doctor there had prescribed some drugs in an attempt to alleviate the problem, but it was obvious they were doing little if anything for a child who was still having six or seven fits a day and had been doing so since she was nine months old.

Of course she had been scanned and tested in every possible way with the hope of finding what was causing the problem. I guess the obvious place to look would be the brain, so the head would be the area which would have received the most attention. But it is this sort of assumption which causes me all too often to suffer that "Deep Frustration", and this turned out to be a typical case. For me, working on the physical body to try to find the source of a problem can be very limiting, but when we step up to the higher frequency energy field which surrounds every living thing, be it the human body, your cat or dog, or the leaves of a tree, we immediately supersede those limits.

Everything in the body is reflected in that energy field, so if there is a group of cells somewhere in a body which has become out of phase with all the others, then the negative energy in that portion of the field, or as it is often referred to, the aura, will create a resistance to the movement of the hand above the body, and the healer will know that his hand has reached the source of the problem in the patient. You will notice I used the word, source, and I can assure you there is a very good reason why I did so. I have long since realised that the place where the problem manifests in the body, is not necessarily the source of the trouble, but is merely the visible symptom, and all too often the medical practitioner considers this to be the area which he should concentrate on in order to remove the problem.

With that thought firmly in our minds, let us go back to the eighteen-month old girl on my couch. The first thing I do with every patient is to visualise the arteries of the body which run from the heart down to the feet. Very often a lot of poison or unwanted dross of some kind will be found in those arteries, so I begin at the left foot and make my way along the leg all the way up to the heart, gradually clearing that dross until I find my hand will run smoothly along the whole area without any resistance to its movement. Only then is it time to move over to the right leg and repeat the process. When this has been completed then the hand goes back to the left foot, and I think to myself, OK, the blood is clear now so I will change frequency and look for any other negative energy above the leg.

This is perhaps the most amazing phenomena which takes place during the healing process. How little we know about this wonderful thing we call the brain. If I set out to clear blood only from the artery in a leg, then that is all that will happen. No other problems in that leg will have any effect on the movement of my hand whatsoever, yet having cleared the blood and changed the frequency of my thought pattern merely by thinking to myself, now I will look for any other negative energy, my hand may suddenly come up against what I often refer to as a brick wall as it approaches perhaps the ankle or the knee, and I know there is a problem there for me to work on. Yet a few moments ago as my hand passed along precisely the same area but with my mind tuned to the frequency of blood alone, there was nothing to suggest there was anything wrong with that ankle or knee.

What a wonderful computer we have, and what a tragedy it is that we have barely begun to understand what we could do with it if only we were more aware of its latent ability waiting for us to recognise it and put it to use. As always I cleared the blood on our little girl, then began to look for any other negative area in the energy field which may be the source of this distressing problem. Nothing was found in the legs as one might expect in this case, so my next move was to work on the torso, starting at the bottom and working my way up to the shoulders. My hand had only travelled a very short distance along the centre of the lower torso when it refused to go any further. Could this be the "SOURCE" of the problem so far away from the brain where it was manifesting to create the many fits she was suffering from? Surely if this was so the medical people who had been working with her these past nine months would have discovered it long ago and done something about it.

But as I worked on this one small area I began to realise exactly what was happening here. I mentally recalled some similar cases I had worked on in the past. Some who had been having epileptic fits, but also others who had been suddenly fainting and just dropping in a heap for no apparent reason. In each of these cases it had finally become obvious to me that I was working on the female area, or in some cases, male organ area, and that the true source of the problem was a simple matter of a hormone imbalance which was affecting the brain.

No wonder all the scanning of the brain had shown nothing amiss in that area, for there was nothing wrong there at all. Some time later when my hand finally reached the head it did not detect any negative energy there whatsoever. All my time and hard work was spent on the female area in this case and I could find no other place in the body where my hand could detect any negative energy at all. How could they have missed this in nine months of tests at the most prestigious children's hospital in the country? Surely they must be aware of what hormones can do to a brain when they become out of balance. It is no secret that some females who finish up in a mental home during the period often referred to as "Change of Life", do so because of a hormone problem, but why are they not aware that the same hormones can affect the brains of people of all ages in different ways.

You may well be asking me what proof I have that this hormone problem I was working on had anything to do with her epileptic fits. The answer to that question came a few days later in the form of a phone call from the child's mother. It went something like this. "Mr Lambert, you are not going to believe this, but since you worked on my little girl she has gone from her usual six or seven fits a day to no more than one or two. It is just wonderful". I told her I could easily believe that because it was no more than a repetition of similar cases I had worked on in the past. I told her that while we had already gained a substantial measure of success, we would need to work on her at least one more time to bring about the complete balancing of the hormones and the total ceasing of the epilepsy and this she agreed to do in the near future.

At this stage the whole plan for her recovery took a turn in a direction that I could never have dreamed of. I had a phone call from a business in Auckland City who make documentaries for our TV stations. The caller told me he had received a request from the main TV station in the country to make a one-hour documentary. They had told him that owing to the rapid increase of the people out there in their interest in alternative medicine and healing etc, they had some money for his firm to make a documentary for them covering the many aspects of these alternatives. It is well to remember that statement concerning the TV people suddenly finding they had some money for this specific purpose, because I am sure that before I finish this story it will become quite clear where this money came from and why.

I told the caller I was not interested in being a part of this documentary because back in 1974 I had made the mistake of taking a TV camera man and a female interviewer to Manila in the Philippines when I took a group of patients with me to visit the Psychic Surgeons. They had taken some wonderful footage of operations being carried out by these healers, using nothing but their hands to open the body and close it again after removing anything from an ulcer to a large cancer growth. But when the resulting tape was shown on TV in NZ, it soon became obvious that it had been doctored in such a way as to make the healers look like fakes and charlatans, and I did not want to be caught like that again.

They assured me it would not be like that this time and they would travel down from Auckland to discuss it with me. They duly arrived next day and spent an hour here telling me what they planned to do. I finally agreed to be a part of it on one condition. I pointed up to the wall where I had a large laminated copy of an extract from the writings of Hippocrates, the same as the one which can be found on page viii of this book. I told them if they would agree to put it on the screen at the time I was doing my demonstration of healing long enough for people to read it, then I was prepared to go along with their proposal. They assured me that would be no problem, and having noticed a copy of my last book You Too Can Heal plus a video of the same name on a shelf beside them, they said they would photograph those and show them on the screen for a few moments so that the viewers would know I had them for sale and it would give me a chance to make a few dollars from the whole project.

As they were leaving, I told them it would be necessary for them to have a good patient in their studio for me to work on the day I travelled to Auckland to do my part. But two days before that was to take place, they rang me to say they had not found a suitable patient and wondered if I knew of anyone I could use. I told them about the little girl who had been in my healing room a few days ago, and as she needed another healing, then perhaps we could do the work at her mother's home. This was all arranged, and we all met there on the due date. Cameras and sound equipment etc were set up and the child was laid on the folding healing couch I had brought with me.

Cameras rolled and I began to work for the second time on our little girl. Sure enough when my hand reached the female area there was still a blockage to be worked on, Thinking the TV people were honest and would be keeping their word concerning the Hippocrates agreement we had made, I started to describe what my hands were doing as they began lifting the negative energy away in order to completely balance the hormones I said "As you can now see on your screen I am pulling and drawing away aches and diverse impurities from the body just as the great father of medicine was doing to his patients nearly two and one half thousand years ago".

What I did not know of course at that stage was the fact that because they had no intention of showing the Hippocrates extract to their viewers, they were going to cut out the piece where I mentioned him. The close up shots they took of my book and video tape suffered the same fate, so instead of making a few dollars selling them as they had suggested I would do, it actually cost me money time and energy travelling to Auckland and back, and I was not even offered a few dollars for my petrol. Not that I would have been the least bit concerned about that if they had just been honest enough to keep their promises.

But much worse to was come. A few days later I had a phone call from the child's mother, she was ringing to tell me that her daughter had not shown any sign of an epileptic fit since the day I had worked on her for TV. Thinking it would be good to have this information given to the viewers when the documentary was shown, I rang the people who made it, but they assured me they had nothing more to do with it. They had been paid for making it, and had sent it on to the TV station. After three toll calls to the station I was finally told that as the documentary was finished they could not add anything to it now. I am sure most readers will know how easy it is to add or delete from a tape these days if you require to do so, and it became very obvious to me that desire was not there.

A few weeks later the big shock came. I was waiting to see the programme which had been advertised for that evening, and I could have cried when I saw what they had done with it. There in front of me was the compere for the one-hour show. She was none other than the well-known comedienne who over a number of years had appeared on TV as Lynn of Tawa. Why would anyone in their right mind use a comedienne as a compere of a documentary about a serious subject such as Alternative Healing unless she was there to make it all look silly. They had not told me she would be the compere, and of course the reason for that became quite obvious the moment I saw her. The makers of the documentary knew only too well that if they had mentioned to me who the compere would be, there was no way they would have been able to talk me into being a part of it.

I watched the programme with several different types of healers and masseurs doing their part while I waited to see how my portion would look on the screen. Then suddenly, there I was, pulling and drawing away from the child aches and diverse impurities in the same way our old friend Hippocrates had done so long ago. But what about the piece where I mentioned him? And what about the close-up of the extract from his writings? Or for that matter where were those shots they took of my book and my tapes? I knew they had taken them because they had done so in my presence. Had this been merely to convince me they would be included in the final tape?

When I had finished what I had to do they did at least have a voice to come on to say that the baby now only has one or two fits a day instead of six or seven and that the mother was understandably grateful. Then our compere came back and made this incredible statement. "Colin believes we all have the potential to be healers, but can we be really certain that it was Colin's magic hands that turned things around for this baby. After all it is not uncommon for small children to grow out of these things as they grow older. So really it is impossible to prove".

Impossible? Only because she had no awareness whatsoever of the hundreds of cases out of the 30,000 or more patients I have had in my healing room who have suddenly "Grown out" of a long standing problem from the very day that I have worked on them. How far can you stretch a coincidence before the theory breaks down? Not satisfied with the growing out of theory, they then introduced a lady doctor and asked her to give her thoughts on the matter. Checking back on the videotape I made of the programme we find this statement. "It is a sad thing and a dangerous thing when a person with a serious illness accepts any alternative therapy which has no possibility of either proper diagnosis or cure, where a cure might well be available in proper scientific medicine".

At the beginning of this chapter I think I said something about deep frustration, and by this time my reader must be beginning to understand at least something of what I meant. If this documentary had been a genuine properly balanced creation, then surely I would have been given the opportunity to reply to the doctor's statement. I would simply have said to her, "You saw me work on that little girl but perhaps you are not aware that the medical people had her for nine months. But even the drugs which the best children's hospital in the country had prescribed for her were doing nothing for the child at all, yet the day after she came to me and I discovered the source of the problem and worked on it, there was an immediate response. How then can you say it is a sad and dangerous thing for someone with a serious illness to try an alternative which has no possibility of proper diagnosis or cure". This of course would have meant giving the viewers a very dangerous thing called "TRUTH", and it had already become very obvious that was the last thing they had any intention of allowing to creep into that documentary.

Some months later I received a lovely card from the grateful mother. Perhaps you would like to know how she felt about what had taken place since she first brought her daughter to me for healing.

"Dear Colin, I am writing to thank you very much for everything you have done for our daughter, (The little girl in the documentary) But even this card doesn't feel like enough. I would love to bring her to see you again and let you see how she is getting on. She still hasn't had any more seizures and it has been almost a year. Her doctor can not believe how she is getting on. He is already talking about stopping her medication if she has not had any more for another twelve months, but I told him that ever since she saw you and been on the TV she hasn't had any more. Thank you very much Colin. She is just a typical two year old little girl now. You have really made a difference in hers and our lives. Thank you."

A short time after receiving this card I called in to see the mother of the child at her home where I had done the healing for the TV, and there was our little girl as her mother put it, running around like any other nearly three-year-old getting into mischief with no sign whatsoever that she had ever been an epileptic. When she told me that although it was nearly a year since she had her last fit, the doctor at Starship was still insisting that she must continue with the drugs he had prescribed, I reckoned it was about time I spoke to him. It had occurred to me that he probably had other patients with similar problems, and if I could only get through to him that he should be looking at a hormone imbalance problem originating in the male or female organ area in these cases instead of scanning the brain where there was nothing wrong apart from being placed under too much stress when the hormones became unbalanced, then there was a much greater chance of the patients being helped.

When I arrived at the hospital he was busy, but after a long wait he finally returned to his office. I introduced myself and began to tell him the reason for my visit. I did not get very far before he became very angry and asked me what I thought I was doing coming to his hospital and wasting his time when I was not even a doctor. I tried to assure him that I was certainly not there to waste his time, but to discuss something with him which I felt sure could be of help to him with other patients with similar problems. His reply to that was to tell me that anything I did had nothing to do with the child not having any more fits. He said it was his drugs which were keeping her from having them, and if he was to stop the drugs then she would start having them again tomorrow.

It was difficult for me to believe that he was really serious in making that statement and asked him would it not be rather much of a coincidence to suggest as he was doing, that after nine months of the drugs doing nothing for the child, they suddenly started to work from the very day I had given her healing. I felt that was bad enough but to say that the fits stopped completely the day after I worked on her the second time for the TV programme was surely stretching coincidence much too far. His anger became even more evident as he pointed to the door and said, "This conversation is at an end. Leave my hospital".

Did I say something about frustration? How else could I feel but frustrated. Surely there can be none so blind as those who do not wish to see. I see again that sign on the wall in my healing room which says it all. "Minds are like parachutes, they only function when they are open". Some time after the documentary was shown I was in Auckland City and called into the office of the firm who made it. I specifically wanted to know why they had used a comedienne as a compere on a serious subject such as the people's health. His answer was really not all that surprising. I felt I already had an answer to that question but I wanted to have the confirmation straight from the horse's mouth as they say. He assured me THEY did not put her on the programme, and mentioned the name of a male TV announcer they wanted to use. But TVNZ who were of course paying them had the last word and insisted that the comedienne must do the job.

You may remember that in the first conversation I had with the makers of the tape, they told me they had received a phone call from TVNZ to say that owing to the rapid increase of the interest of the people in alternative healing they had some money there for their firm to make a one hour documentary. Looking back now on all the evidence I have presented here, it should not be too difficult to work out just who it was who was worried enough about that interest to suddenly provide a few thousand dollars for a documentary. The great majority of the patients who come to me do so in desperation just as that mother had brought her child to me after nine months of tests and drugs had failed to have any effect owing to the fact that the medics had not found the SOURCE of the problem. Each time this happens it means that the patient no longer needs to continue to visit the doctor and that creates two rather drastic results. The doctor, the member of the Medical Association no longer has any money coming into his pocket, but perhaps even more important is the fact that he is no longer writing out any prescriptions for the drugs etc to be supplied by the multi-million dollar drug companies.

Need I say more? As they might say in court, I rest my case and leave it for you to decide where you think the money suddenly came from for that documentary. Perhaps it is just a coincidence that I happened to pick up the newspaper this morning and saw a large headline right across the top of the page. "Australia takes on drug firms." What may become Australia's largest class action has been launched against the European drug companies accused of conspiring to fleece Australians of millions of dollars by overcharging for vitamins. Virtually every Australian has been paying too much for basic food items to feed the greed of company executives in Switzerland, Germany and France said Bernard Murphy of the law firm Maurice, Blackburn, Cashman.

His firm has begun proceedings against F Hoffman, La Roche, BASF-AG and Rhone Poulenc, SA on behalf of Australian companies and a Melbourne woman. The legal action comes after Hoffman La Roche this year pleaded guilty in the United States to orchestrating a worldwide conspiracy to inflate the price of some vitamins. It agreed to pay a fine of $US 500 million - the largest ever in a US criminal case.

Greed, money, power. You, the people need to become aware of the danger you face from these three. Realise that the very last thing you are likely to be presented with willingly is that evasive thing called truth. If you want to find that then look at what you are being told, then take an even better look at what you are deliberately not being told, for this is where you will find truth, hidden behind a smokescreen of words which are presented to you to confuse and to lead you away from that all important truth. It has been well said that the truth will set you free. Seek it diligently, for it is there waiting for those who will make enough effort to find it.

Late last year a lady handed me a long list of very abbreviated notes copied from her diary over the past two years. They concerned her eighteen-year-old daughter, who, in 1996 began fainting and consequently became a long-term patient of her doctor. She listed every visit to the doctor, every ride in an ambulance, and made some mention of the amount of money it had cost her for specialist fees. This is a very long list, and I do not wish to bore you by copying all of it, but I do want to give you some idea of the difference between orthodox medical practise, and what is so vaguely referred to as "Alternative", so I will just offer you a few extracts from it.

It begins with "Fainting began September 1996, Doctors thought she would grow out of it".

Taken half a dozen times from school after fainting.

Feb '97. Specialist, Neurologist. $ 225.00.
Migraines diagnosed. Prescribed Paramax.
Jan '97. Blacked out at skating.
March. Fainted at school. Doctor called.
April. Blacked out on footpath. Doctor.
Taken by ambulance to Thames. In hospital four days.
Three more blackouts and doctor called during April.
29th April. EEG Auckland. $225.00.
May, Blackouts on four dates. Thames Hospital.
Paediatrician one day. Hospital heart monitor four days later.
The list goes on in similar fashion through June, July and August.

About this time the mother took her daughter to see a spinal specialist, thinking the problem may be caused in that area. He examined the spine but decided there was no sign of any problem there. He then did a very strange thing. He suggested she take her daughter back to Waihi and to ask for an appointment with a Mr Lambert as he felt he would be able to sort out the problem for her. The mothers reply was, "Oh, but we live just across the road from him".

I have had a lot of proof over the years of that old saying, "A prophet is without honour in his own country". Not that I am suggesting for one moment that I am a prophet, but I am sure you will know what I mean when I tell you that of all the many thousands of people who visited my healing room over the last twenty-five years or more, very few of those were living in Waihi. They have travelled from every corner of NZ and they have flown in from areas as far apart as Australia, Hawaii, and Holland, but rarely do I see a local.

Back with our 18 year-old girl, we find her finally laying on my couch with a very anxious mother sitting on a chair watching the proceedings. She informed me that a specialist in Auckland had just told her that they had carried out every possible test on her daughter over the past months, and nothing had shown up which would suggest there was anything wrong with her. His final words were, "I think it must be just stress".

How many times have I heard that word used by someone who has come to my room in desperation after the medical people have failed to find the source of their problem? I have long since lost count, but I do know it has been a considerable number. It would appear to be a stock phrase for someone who is loath to admit he or she cannot find the source of the problem in the patient.

I began my work as usual by clearing the blood and then said, "Now we will come back again and look for any other negative energy which may suggest the source of your daughters problem". My hand had barely started to move up the torso when it refused to go any further no matter how hard I pushed it. It was as though I had suddenly come up against a solid wall and there was no way it would move. I remember saying "How could they miss this in all those months of tests? I couldn't miss this if I was riding past on a fast horse". Perhaps a bit of an overstatement I agree, but I felt quite shocked that here beneath my hand was such an obvious negative area which would almost certainly be the cause of all her distress over such a long period of time, yet the best medical people in the country had failed to find it.

How could this be? For me of course there was one very simple answer. The fact that orthodox medics work on the very low and very limiting frequency level of the physical body, but a magnetic healer has stepped up to the much higher frequency of the energy force which surrounds it, and in doing so immediately supersedes many of those limits. It was quite clear that my hand had stopped over the female area of the body which meant that once again we had a simple matter of a hormone imbalance to contend with.

As it turned out this one was not quite as simple as I had expected it to be. If we look again at that long list her mother gave me, we find that although there was some improvements, there were still a few more blackouts and a couple of visits to a doctor over the next few months. However, as the patient only had such a short distance to walk to my healing room, she came over several times for me to work on her again during that time, and although I had to work on the area several times, I did notice that the pressure against my hand was becoming less on each occasion, and I worked a shorter time to clear it.

Now it is more than a year since it has been necessary for her to visit me, and her mother assures me she is fine. How can I ever get through to people who have for many years been trained to follow a particular path in their endeavours, the fact that there is an alternative one which will take them to the destination they are seeking infinitely more quickly and accurately.

3. DOORS BEGIN TO OPEN

It is quite some time now since I decided that perhaps I too needed to follow a different path. I do not mean a different path to the one I have been pursuing very successfully for many years in order to heal the sick, but a different way of breaking through the barrier which the medical fraternity has built around themselves and their very powerful organisation. With this in mind, I theorised that if I could teach enough students the art of Magnetic Healing, then perhaps when doctors found that Mr Jones and Mrs Smith were no longer visiting the surgery, and on enquiry discovered that it was because they were no longer ill simply because they had visited a healer, then maybe they would become worried enough to start looking at something which they had previously considered not to be worth a second thought.

Much of the rest of this book will tell the story of the results of that decision and will bring into print some of the exciting circumstances by which they were brought about. I am of course, not the only one who is dedicating their time and effort towards bringing this about, so what I want to do here is to record something of the co-ordination of many factors and many people which are together slowly helping to bring this to fruition. Many times in my lectures or workshops around the world I have pointed out to my audience that I have been attempting to do to the best of my ability for the past thirty years, two separate achievements.

One has been to heal the sick in body mind and soul, and judging by the results of that work it would seem as though that task has been reasonably well performed. But the other one has been infinitely more difficult. It is what I call "Educating the Educated", and to a large extent what I have discovered in trying to do this is the fact that if you hit your head on a brick wall it hurts. But what I really do want to tell you is that as each year goes by the wall appears to be getting softer, and it does not hurt so much when I hit it. In other words I am saying, on an ever increasing number of occasions the opposition to what I have to say to educated people is softening in many quarters, and scientifically or medically minded people are beginning to take a second look at methods of healing which in the not very distant past they would have relegated to the loony bin.

One only needs to look at Acupuncture. It is not many years ago that Western medics looked on that as some strange belief the Chinese had, but today it is almost universally accepted as a legitimate method of healing and has actually been taken on by numerous doctors as an adjunct to their normal treatment. I well remember one particular time when I was spending a few days in a New Zealand city lecturing and teaching. I was introduced one morning to a Chinese doctor, and as he was suffering from very bad headaches he asked me if I would work on him to try to bring some relief. This I did for quite some time, and after I had finished I sat back on a chair to rest. The doctor was still laying on the couch relaxing, but after a short time he sat up and said, "You know Colin, I understand what you are all about and what you are doing, but I also know why most doctors would not even begin to comprehend what has just been taking place here." He went on to explain that like any other doctor he had spent six or seven years training and all through that time he could barely ever remember hearing the word "Energy" mentioned.

But not all that long ago he had decided to take a course in acupuncture and was now using that method in conjunction with his normal medical services. He told me that during this training the word energy was the one he would have heard more often than any other, along with such words as Chakra, meridians and Lifeforce. They were informed that when something has gone wrong with a body it usually means that there is a blockage somewhere which is inhibiting the natural flow of the Lifeforce to a particular group of cells, so in a sense this group of cells is virtually dying. No cells can remain in good working order without the life giving energy flowing through to them. So they were shown how to discover what one might call a dam which was impeding the flow of that energy, and were then instructed how to use very fine needles to break down that dam to allow the energy to once again flow through to the cells and rebuild them, thereby allowing the body to become what we call well again.

But it was his last statement which really hit me as being something which I had never expected to come from a doctor. He said, "That is exactly what you are doing, but without any needles. You are just using your hands". What an enlightening statement. Not that he was really telling me anything I didn't already know, but I found it to be very satisfying to discover that here at last was one doctor who did understand, and I felt that maybe some of this different attitude towards alternative methods of healing must surely rub off on some of his colleagues as he works and speaks with them.

Since that time I have had the pleasure of discussing my work with several very open minded doctors, and although the majority may still be at least very wary and a certain number totally opposed to any change whatsoever from their long cherished beliefs, the number whose parachutes are finally opening continues to grow ever more rapidly as the months and years go by. I now feel the time is approaching when those stubborn ones who flatly refuse to even consider there may be something of value to be found outside the normally accepted methods will find themselves being left behind and isolated from those who are following the much more exciting and rewarding trend toward what has been for all too long labelled as alternative.

Perhaps of all the experiences I have had in this regard since I wrote "You Too Can Heal" six years ago took place in August of last year when I was in Vermont USA. I spent about a week staying with my wonderful organiser Lisa and her husband in their lovely big log cabin home. Long before I ever arrived she had made arrangements for a public meeting in a hall at the local school plus workshops in the very large room at her home. But I was thrilled to find that she had also organised something else which had the potential of being a very interesting and rewarding experience. She told me that a Doctor Anderson had a one hour programme one morning each week on a radio station in a nearby city. The programme was titled "Health and Longevity" and sometimes he would interview a guest on different aspects of medical matters. The Friday I was to be in the area had been set aside for me to be his guest on that day.

As we sat in the studio waiting for the signal to begin our part of the mornings broadcasting, he asked me what sort of questions he should put to me when we went on air. I suggested that probably the most appropriate one to begin with would be to request me to describe to his thousands of listeners in the city and beyond what I have called Magnetic Healing. I am well aware that many people have never heard the name mentioned, and I find there are some who think that I use magnets, and are not aware that everything I do is done with bare hands, and no "props" whatsoever. After duly introducing me to his listeners and giving them a short rundown of some of the things I had been doing at home and around the world over the past thirty years he finally put the question to me. My reply went something like this.

"I could answer that question in my own words, but what I am going to do is to let someone else do it for me. I am sure as a medical person you will have heard of this man even though it is the best part of two and one half thousand years since he was here in the flesh. I am of course referring to none other than the one which the medical profession refers to as the "Father of medicine" and whose Hippocratic oath they sign".

At this stage I reached into my pocket and brought out a copy of the extract from his writings which I mentioned in chapter two and read it to the listeners. When I had finished I pointed out that the reason why I had done it this way was because I did not consider I could have done it any better myself. The way in which he described feeling the heat oozing from his hands and applying it to the sick in order to be able to pull and draw away aches and diverse impurities was a perfect explanation of the way in which I had worked on my thousands of patients. I then told him and his listeners that there was only one thing which I did not understand about all this. And that was the fact that while medical people in general considered Hippocrates to be the father of medicine and signed his Hippocratic oath, the great majority of them would scoff at one who follows in his footsteps today by working in precisely the same manner as this great man did so long ago.

The rest of my hour on his programme was taken up with some very interesting discussion on the merits of alternative healing in general and a description of some of the more dramatic healings I have had the pleasure and privilege of performing on some very desperate patients during my many years as a healer. Mention was then made of the public meeting where I would be demonstrating this work in a hall at the local high school, and the fact that I would also be holding several workshops where I would be showing groups of around twenty people at a time how they could become healers and channels for the Loveforce.

But more was to come. Much more. When we went off air the good doctor told me he was a little worried about a problem which his wife was suffering from, and wondered if I would be prepared to come to his surgery at five pm after his last patient had left and check her out. Needless to say I didn't need to give much thought to that request before deciding on the answer, with the result that a few minutes after five I found myself standing beside a couch in the doctors surgery running my hands through the energy field of his wife. Surely this must be the sort of thing that a healers dreams are made of, but not something which he or she dares to expect to become reality. To see him step up to the couch at my request, and move his hands through his wife's energy field, then suddenly find them beginning to shake as they approached the area where I had indicated there was a problem was an added bonus. I am sure that little episode came to an end with three very happy people heading off to a restaurant for an evening meal.

During the next few days Lisa and I travelled twice into the city. One trip was to be a part of the seven a.m. morning news at the TV station and the other was to attend a book signing at the very large Barnes and Noble bookstore where fifty or sixty people lined up to hear me speak about my work for about half an hour, and then demonstrate Magnetic Healing on the shoulder of the husband of the manager. I then sat at the table and signed about twenty five copies of "You Too Can Heal" as people bought them.

Saturday was public meeting day, and around one hundred and twenty people gathered in the High School Auditorium. After Dr Anderson spoke about his interest in alternative medicine he introduced me, and I then began to show about fifty colour slides on a large screen. These slides consisted of many different aspects of the importance of understanding that there is nothing throughout an endless Universe but energy. Energy in its many forms and frequencies of vibration, and my experiences over the years have taught me that until Earthman becomes aware of this and realises that he must leave behind him what we commonly refer to as "science" and gain a whole new understanding of the science of the higher frequency energies and put them to use, we will continue to pollute Mother Earth and her environs in a way which can only be spelt out as disaster.

It is not too late. Nature has a wonderful capacity to rebuild herself, but we must be prepared to give her a hand instead of continuing to show her that in our greed, our selfishness and our boundless ignorance we are determined to make it impossible for her to do so. We must realise that she is our mother, the great provider, and if she becomes ill, then we follow in her footsteps. The ozone layer, the warming of the planet, the pollution of land, sea and air. All of these and many more are the result of that mixture of greed and ignorance.

Judging by the prolonged applause which followed the showing of the slides and the explanation I gave in conjunction with them, I gathered the audience had enjoyed what they had seen and heard, and I felt that the time and energy expended in bringing the information to them had been well rewarded.

Strange that at this time in my writing I should just happen to pick up this mornings newspaper to see if there was anything of particular interest in it, for the first headline I saw said, “Breast milk check coming”. The report went on to say, “The Government will set out to find if breast milk in this country is contaminated after a British study found more than three hundred and fifty chemicals from substances such as perfume, suntan lotion, and pesticides in mothers milk. Some of the contaminants identified are known to have the ability to cause cancer, and some are able to impair the immune system. Other substances found were known to interfere with the normal function of the bodies hormones”. “Hormones”. That word sounded all too familiar. A nine months old girl having epileptic fits. An eighteen year old young woman continually fainting. And both of them completely cleared simply by working to balance the hormones. Coincidence, or interesting fact.

The following day the doctor and his wife attended my second workshop for the day and sat with about eighteen others in the lovely big room at Lisa's home. When it was time for the doctors wife to come up beside the couch and feel the area of negative energy in the patients aura as several others had already done, I was very pleased to see that she was experiencing quite a lot of resistance to the movement of her hand as she approached it. After some effort she managed to cup it together, and, turning to her right away from me, she threw it away. Many times I have seen tears flowing freely from the eyes of someone who has just had this experience for the first time, and although this is not quite the description I would give in this case, it was clear that she was having difficulty in stemming their flow as she leaned on my shoulder for a few moments while she gained her composure before returning to her seat beside her husband.

A ripple of laughter ran through the room as I said to her, “My word, the way you were working on that patient, you will be daddies little helper from now on”. This feature of tears and bewilderment for someone who feels the energy for the first time and realises that he or she really does have the ability to place their hands over an ailing body and to remove the pain and suffering from that body is a common attribute of my teaching work. Something happens inside at this time. Some say they did not feel anything in their hands as they approached the problem area, but do complain that they experienced a strange feeling in their shoulders, their stomach, or maybe their head. I tell them I don’t care if their big toe wiggles, as long as something different happens somewhere in their body as their hand approaches the negative energy. There were many that day in the two classes I held, who showed by their reactions that they were having a strong response to that energy, and I was particularly happy to see our doctor friend was among them.

Another strange thing which takes place at this time is the rapidly changing colour of the hands of the student. While their hand is passing along above the body in an area where there is nothing wrong, the hands stay their normal colour, but for most, as soon as they begin to enter the problem area and come up against the resistance it creates, they begin to go red, and some go so deep in colour that they take on an almost purple hue. I have often thought that I would like to be able to ask a doctor if he or she could give me any explanation of this strange phenomena, especially in view of the fact that so many doctors in the past who I have approached concerning my work, have chased me away with some comment like, "There is no way I would ever believe you could do anything by waving your hands over a body" as one lady doctor had said to me.

Here was my chance at last to ask that question. But of course here we had one of those all too rare doctors who had the good fortune to have an open mind, so that the question did not cause him any concern whatsoever. He went on to explain to the group his considered opinion, and while I cannot now remember his exact words, I do know he said something about the corpuscles filling with blood very rapidly at that time. If we are doing nothing by "Waving our hands over a body" then will someone please tell me why it always only happens when the hands are over the area on the patient where the problem lies. And remember that always the healer has been told nothing of what the patient is suffering from, so how does he know to tell his hands to go red just in the right spot which is nearly always confirmed later as being the very place the patient has his problem. Surely there can be none so blind as those who do not wish to see. Yes, minds are like parachutes, they really do only work when they are open, and in this case it was a great pleasure and privilege to be able to work with one whose parachute was wide open and ready for use. May there be many more of them as the years roll by, and may many suffering people on Planet Earth gain new health, hope and upliftment as the inhibiting levels of ignorance are slowly swept aside to make way for the enlightenment which will follow.

Doctor Valerie Hunt, Professor Emeritus at UCLA (University of California in Los Angeles) has stated that official acceptance of subtle energies and energy medicine is just around the corner for Western Medical science, and says it will follow the inevitable three-step pattern of all great innovative ideas. First it will be ridiculed, then it will be tolerated, and finally it will be held as self evident truth by everybody. Over my years of experience in this field, I have certainly seen more than enough of the ridiculing, have watched a gradual movement towards tolerance, with a slowly increasing number of scientific and medical people taking their first step in that direction, but at this stage I still await with bated breath the time when the latter will become fact, and healers drawing on the Universal Energy to bring new health to ailing bodies will be as readily accepted as prescribing drugs is today.

In an excellent book "The Common Touch" written by Tom Harpur, we find this interesting statement. "It will come as news to many in North America that there are now at least three general practise surgeries in England with Spiritual Healers paid by the government under the National Health Plan. A growing number of British doctors now refer their patients to healers at the healer's treatment rooms. A dozen or so doctors to date have declared they are developing their own innate healing powers. Two hospital pain centres and two hospital cancer centres have healers on the staff of the health team. Some fifteen hundred healers have had access to British hospitals".

About two years ago I had the privilege of organising some meetings in several areas of New Zealand for a Spiritual healer who came to visit from England. She was Lorraine Ham, a healer who for ten years has been a member of Britain's National Federation of Spiritual Healers. She works as a healer at a clinic in Ottley, Yorkshire, with eight doctors and four nurses. In addition, she and another woman healer visit regularly in local hospitals.

She said that when she was first hired by the team of physicians at Ottley they only sent her the most difficult cases, "their failures", a lot of whom were taking long-term medications and suffering from multiple psychological problems. All eight doctors still refer this type of patient to her, but they now also send her the less seriously ill. What I do is complimentary to what the doctors do, not an alternative. It gives the patient an option as well. She says that in Britain anyway, we are taught to have a stiff upper lip and to suppress our emotions to the point where many patients facing painful therapies or terminal prognoses are lying there paralysed by terror and unable to get release. The nurses often worry about these people. They want to help but very often they can not reach them. In these cases a healer can help unblock all this emotional energy and ease the pain.

I have no idea how many times I have been working on a very sick female on my couch when they have suddenly burst into tears. I tell them,

"That's good love just let it all go. You have been bottling it up too long. Let it go." And they do. But it is always an enjoyable experience for me when I see them walk out my door and say something like, "I feel so light. It is like I am floating above your concrete." And I sometimes think that maybe it is just as well my wife does not see the many who just want to cry on my shoulder or give me a big hug before they leave. It is as though they are saying I am stuck for words to say thank you, but I want you to know how I feel about what you have done for me. I have not spent a lot of time in doctors' surgeries, but I doubt that you would see that sort of emotional outpouring of relief very often. They are more likely to be hanging onto the prescription for some drug the doctor has written out for them than hanging onto the doctor.

I titled this chapter, "Doors begin to open" and I am very happy to be able to say there is a very good reason for that. I have already mentioned one or two of them, but let us take a look at some of the changes in this regard around the world, particularly for my readers who may be quite unaware that this movement toward a more general recognition of the many complimentary methods of healing is gathering momentum at an ever increasing rate. For instance in 1993 I cut an article from a newspaper which was referring to a report of a study of Holistic Medical treatment which appeared in the New England journal of Medicine. It explained Holistic therapies as those which treated the whole person, physically and psychologically rather than just treating a diseased part.

I must admit I was a little surprised but very pleased to see that a journal of medicine was prepared to point out this difference between the normal method of prescribing some medicine in an attempt to reverse the problem in the body and what I sometimes describe as the body, mind and soul healing of complimentary treatment. The article went on to say that the study had found about one in three Americans seeks out some form of Holistic medical treatment each year, and the cost of that care rivals what patients pay for more conventional medical therapy. The study found that an estimated US$ twelve billion was paid out on unconventional therapy in 1990, the year it was conducted, of which US$ ten billion was paid out of pocket by individuals. By comparison US$ twelve billion was spent out of pocket on all hospital stays. And that was nine years ago, so I would not like to try to guess what the figures would look like today.

Another clipping I saved since 1996 makes interesting reading. It was headlined, "Traditional Healers Return" and went on to say that traditional medicines used for centuries in Asia and Africa are experiencing a boom in the industrialised countries of the West according to the World Health Organisation. Acupuncture, Herbal medicine and traditional healers and midwives are also resisting the pressure of Western Science in their countries of origin, with some eighty per cent of the world's population having recourse to such methods. In the past two decades they have found favour in Europe and North America despite sophisticated modern treatments and the power of the pharmaceutical lobbies. A third of adult Americans used alternative healing methods, while in Britain the Consumers Association found that one in four of its members had consulted non-conventional practitioners in 1991, compared with one in seven in 1985.

Statements like these surely bare out what I have said concerning the gradual movement toward a more holistic understanding of the body and the need to treat it as such. Coming a little more up to date, I have in front of me a newspaper dated March '98 and it has a large picture of a woman looking at a rubber model with many needles stuck in it. The caption underneath says it all.

Dr Joan Campbell of Auckland demonstrates the instruments of Chinese Acupuncture on a rubber model showing the body's acupuncture points. She will take a team of doctors and nurses to China for a four week study tour which is sponsored by the Asia 2,000 Foundation and is part of the graduate diploma course at Auckland Institute of Technology. She says you should arm yourself with the skills you have to experience the culture. Acupuncture is one of the most rapidly growing forms of medical treatment here she says. Chinese traditional medicine never separates body from mind and looks into the root cause and symptoms.

Perhaps my younger readers will not consider the foregoing as being anything particularly remarkable, for you will have grown up with the word "Acupuncture" being pretty much a part of Western language and acceptance, but I am sure that my more elderly ones will remember as I do, a time not so many years ago when it was looked on as being some strange belief which the people of China had talked them into, and of course with no scientific basis whatsoever. That information was printed as I have said in March '98, but let us take a look at one year later in March '99. Dr William Fair thought he knew all there was to know about cancer. But it was only when he got it himself that he made the discovery that could change the way we treat the disease for ever.

One morning last month Dr Fair downed the Chinese herbal remedy he believes has helped to keep his cancer at bay for eighteen months. Then he went to give a lecture to his colleagues on the value of meditation, prayer and vitamins in fighting cancer. What makes this so remarkable is that Dr Fair is a leading cancer surgeon at one of Americas most high-tech specialist cancer hospitals, Memorial Sloan-Kettering in New York where the merest mention of herbs or meditation is heresy. Two years ago Dr Fair was himself an arch exponent of scientific medicine and unquestionably one of the team."

A common question I get from patients who come to my healing room with a serious problem is a simple, "Why me?" Sometimes they are obviously very upset and consider they have been handed a very raw deal. They point out that they have lived a pretty good life and tried not to harm anyone, and then they get hit with this terrible thing. Life seems to be so unfair they tell me. While I can understand very well why people feel this way at a time like this, I can look back on many of these cases and realise that very often this sickness was no accident. Just as Dr Fair had to be faced with the very problem himself which he had been trying to help others with before he would consider there may be a better way of doing it, so I have seen many of those who have come to me for physical healing, make unbelievable changes in their lives. Some of them have been so busy working and storing up material gains in the form of money, fancy cars or whatever, that they have not had time to give any thought whatsoever to their Spiritual development.

Then suddenly they find themselves sitting around with a lot of time on their hands. This becomes time to think, and perhaps for the first time in their life they begin to question and ask themselves what life is really all about. Why am I here? What am I supposed to be doing? Is this problem I have going to end it? What have I really achieved by being here anyway? I know these are some of the questions which are running around, usually in circles of complete confusion in their minds, because these are the same questions they put to me. Apart from answering them to the best of my ability while I am working on them, I very often sell them one of my books. On a number of occasions I have received a phone call the next morning from yesterday's visitor jokingly complaining that she wished she had not bought that book from me. When I ask her why she is saying that, she tells me it is because she hardly got any sleep last night owing to the fact that she could not put it down.

When this happens, I feel a little bit like the keen fisherman who holds his rod for a long time with nothing happening. Then suddenly there is a mighty tug on his line and he knows his patience has been rewarded. A fish has been hooked. And when someone goes to the trouble to ring me with that sort of "complaint" then I know that, like the fish, that one has been hooked, and their life will never be quite the same. But they had to become ill first before they could find the time, something they kept telling themselves they never had, to sit back and take a long hard look at what they were doing with their life. Are they doing what they came here to do? Are they really achieving anything of lasting value? Have they learned anything which they can take with them when the time comes for them to step aside from this very temporary home we call the body and return to what I often refer to as the "Real World", the world of Spirit from whence they came when they stepped into that physical body at the point of time which we refer to as birth.

As the Bible puts it, the soul incarnate and the soul discarnate. The same living soul whether it be incarnate within the physical form for a short period on the Earthplane in order to learn certain lessons you cannot learn without a physical body to work through, or that, at least for most of us, invisible form sometimes referred to as Spirit. I say for most of us, simply because I have had many people over the years describe to me Spirit forms they have seen working with me or just standing watching, and although I do not "See" in this way myself, I am well aware that when we work in this way with the higher frequency energies in order to bring health and hope to our fellow beings in need, we are never alone. All the help you could ever need is waiting for you to request it. "Ask and thou shalt receive" is a very good piece of advice to remember.

This is one of those times in my writing when I suddenly realise my pen has not stopped flowing for some time and the writing is beginning to scrawl a little as the pen continues to flow across the page. Then I think to myself, " What am I writing about here anyway? So it is time to rest the hand for a short time and go back a little and check. After all, the heading on this chapter was "Doors begin to open", and I was writing about the medical people changing their attitude towards alternative methods of healing, so how come I have switched off onto another line and started writing about people who come for healing etc.

Yes, of course. I see it now. It does make sense after all. Maybe my invisible scribe at this time could see that "Opening Doors" was not just something which needed to be done for medics, but for all those who have a desire to seek the eternal truths and in so doing, change their lives around for the better, and thereby achieve the goals which they had set out to fulfil before they ever left the Spirit World to become clothed for a short period of time in human flesh. Perhaps he was looking way ahead to the time when these words my pen is forming have become an actual book, and some reader just needed what has been written on the last page or two. Maybe it is someone who has just been informed that they have a serious medical problem and are at a loss to know how to face a future which has suddenly been darkened by a heavy cloud of uncertainty which has been thrown over them. Perhaps the foregoing will help to lift that cloud a little and allow a greater measure of the light of understanding to come streaming into their life.

Having said all that, let us now return to the original purpose for writing this chapter, the opening of doors to allow the converging of orthodox and alternative. A melding of the two that all may gain from this unison. June 1996 saw me visiting Vancouver in Canada. While I will expect to be recording some interesting facts about that trip a little later in another chapter, I want to mention at this stage something which took place on just one of the days I spent there. On this particular morning I was having my breakfast when my host handed me the latest edition of the Vancouver Sun for me to read. He had seen the large headline at the top of the page and knew I would be keen to read it. "East Meets West at Vancouver Hospital".

And of course, with a headline like that, he was right. That was one paper they never got to use for lighting the fire or wrapping some rubbish in. That one came home in my suitcase, and was put into a large envelope with a number of other interesting pieces of information in readiness for the time when I would finally get that inner feeling that this was the time to bring it all together and present it to my eagerly awaiting readers.

The story began with these words. "A respected physician has convinced the facility to open a privately funded institute to research treatments such as Acupuncture and homoeopathy". Elaine Stevens never thought she would see the day. Vancouver Hospital, that bastion of high-tech health care is opening an institute for complementary medicine this fall and likes the idea of having Stevens plant a herb garden at the front door. "Its fabulous" Stevens, a herbalist said in her west side backyard where herbs such as lovage and ladies-mantle grow in lush profusion. "We are looking at a major shift in thinking". What is practised at Vancouver hospital is Western medicine, also called conventional, orthodox or allopathic. But its officials are prepared to have the $400 million a year institution look seriously at herbs, acupuncture, homeopathy and other disciplines that are considered complimentary or alternative all because a Vancouver doctor convinced them it was time.

Paediatric specialist Dr Wah Jun Tze is the reason why, this October, Vancouver Hospital will open the Tze–Chi institute for complimentary and alternative medicine on Twelfth Avenue. Tze has managed to get this unique synthesis of Western and Eastern medicine off the ground partly because his conventional medicine credentials are impeccable. While visiting China several times over the last ten years, Tze began to harbour a sneaking sympathy for the country's age old healing traditions. He saw a Chinese mushroom extract help an acquaintance recover from cancer that would be considered terminal in the west. And in Vancouver he saw acupressure, massage and herbal patches give his dentist wife more relief from lower back pain than conventional treatments ever provided. "Traditional medicine has years and years of history" said Tze. "Common sense says there is possibly something there. There is no question in my mind that we have an obligation to look at it".

Now most other major Lower Mainland hospitals are supporting his institute. The British Columbia Cancer Agency, the University of BC Medical School and even the provinces conservative college of physicians and surgeons are considering lending the institute their support. Dr Thomas Handly, Registrar of the Doctors College said, "It is being presented with the sponsorship of a reputable medical scientist. We see the very distinct possibility of this fulfilling a very good function". Dr Rogers, a senior Vancouver general practitioner known for his open minded attitude to other modes of healing, said today's well informed consumers are driving the demand for alternatives".

I kid you not. These really are statements coming from the mouths of well respected medical men and women, and they no longer appear to be concerned that their names are attached publicly to thoughts, ideas and beliefs which only a few short years ago would have been looked at by the hierarchy of the medical profession as hearsay. Yes my friend, doors are opening. Some of them are barely more than ajar, but others are slowly opening wider and wider as each month and each year slides by, while a few are already preparing to place the welcome mat beneath the gaping hole where a barrier with something like "Orthodox Believers Only" written on it once stood.

I have long since learned that there is no point in saying something unless you are somebody, and at this stage in the eyes of many medical or scientific people I am nobody. Perhaps if I had Doctor or Professor in front of my name or a string of letters after it then I would not be chased away when I approach one of these as I was at Starship Hospital as mentioned in chapter two, not to mention several other similar occasions over several years.

In a little book printed in Bombay with the title of "Handbook of Magnetic Cure", we find some interesting statements such as the following. "What is most needed now is that physicians who are engaged in the practise of medicine should fairly investigate the method of curing disease by psychological power, or vital magnetism, and when they have ascertained that they themselves possess the latent power in any degree, to be courageous enough to cultivate it, when by so doing they can benefit their fellow beings". I can go along with that statement 100%, and from what I have already told you about the doctor in Vermont who came to my workshop to learn the techniques of Magnetic Healing it is clear that a few are heading in this direction, and I applaud that, but another extract from the same book gives one little to cheer over.

"We have heard of physicians in whom the Magnetic Power had been developed, and so acknowledged to their patients, yet when one of these was suffering in the extreme, and their prescriptions failed to afford relief, refused to call into the service of their art this natural gift. The reason given was that it was not according to their school of practise, and they did not want to do anything in the way of treating disease by this method even if they knew it would give relief.".

In one instance, where the physician himself was sick, and the benefit of Magnetic treatment was offered, he refused it, not only on the ground already stated, but also because it conflicted with his religious belief, alleging that if he received benefit from its use it would help the cause, and he would rather die than employ a professional healer. Oh well, I guess you can't win them all. We just have to push on and keep our eyes open for that steadily growing number of welcome mats that are slowly but surely being placed beneath the doors which lead into what was considered to be the most Holy of Holies, and I say this in both a medical and religious sense.

Since I wrote those last few lines I have had a lovely nights sleep and a new day has dawned. Ever since I started my healing work I realised that when you are prepared to spend your time and energy and effort in pursuit of health and happiness for your brothers and sisters of the planet, then you are never alone. A guiding hand points the way and your life becomes full of what the uninitiated would probably refer to as coincidences. This morning was no exception. My mail box was bursting with mail from several areas, and my first thought when I saw it all was, "Oh no. Just when I thought I had a free day to continue with my writing".

I guess maybe I am just a slow learner and should by now have realised that nothing ever happens by accident in this work. Last night I reckoned I had just about completed this chapter concerning the doors which were beginning to open, and was giving some thought to the direction I should take in chapter four. Amongst the mail today was one of those official Post Office bubble bags which had been sent to me from the South Island of NZ. Among its contents was a three hour videotape, and I reckoned the last thing I wanted to do today was to sit and watch a video. But a label attached to the tape said, "This is a tape which contains an item about magnetic healing. Thought you might like to copy it and send it back". Oh well, I did so much want to get on with writing that book today, but if she wants this sent back then I expect I had better take a look at it and see if there is anything there worth copying.

It was well into the afternoon before I finally sat down at my desk to begin penning these words. You see there was a letter from a different part of the South Island which contained a cheque for a copy of my first book "Why" and one of my fourth book "You Too Can Heal" plus one of my video tapes. So that had to be attended to first before I was able to sit down and view the tape. What the sender of the tape had not mentioned was the fact that the three or four minute item about magnetic healing was at least two and one hours into a three hour tape. Every now and then I became so disgusted with some of the content that I would switch it onto fast forward and watch the programme flashing by without sound, but slow enough to allow me to see if anything interesting turned up.

And then it happened. There we were at a seminar where there were several people demonstrating different methods of healing, so the tape was immediately put back to the normal play position. There was a man using a most unusual method of healing by vibrations which he created with his mouth close up to the patients body. A new method for me, but as I know there is nothing but energy in its many forms and frequencies of vibration, and that many of these vibrations, whether it be through the medium of sounds as this one was demonstrating, or colour such as some use, then it was certainly not for me to condemn in any way whatsoever because it was not the way I work. I always say it is not the method you use which is important, but whether the patient has been healed. That is the only thing of any real importance in your healing room, because that is what he or she came in the door for.

But then it really happened, and I knew why this tape had to arrive today and not tomorrow when I would have finished this chapter about opening doors and gone onto something else. The commentator said something like "Just around the corner from the crystal display we find a lady with a most unusual gift. She runs her hands over ailing bodies and after discovering where the problem is, she begins healing". But let us now take the exact words as they come from the tape. When asked to tell the viewers what she was doing she gave this reply. "Energy comes out of my hands. It is not magic. It is electromagnetic energy. This has been studied by scientists. I utilise energy because energy works the quickest".

Commentator "You would never guess what she does for a living. DOCTOR Susan Coles is a certified plastic surgeon. That is what she does for a living. She has nine years of medical training." The next scene moved to a hospital where Dr Coles was seen removing a ruptured silicon breast implant. When she had it all away and the normal operation as any other surgeon would perform was completed we were shown something which I had previously thought I would be very lucky to see in my lifetime. She began moving her hands above the body of the patient in precisely the way that I have done on so many thousands of patients both here and around the world during those wonderful last twenty five years. She said she was moving her hands through what she called a force-field. It is as if you have put your hand into an electrical magnetic field. The interviewer asked her if there would be a difference if she healed only one side of the chest, and the doctor assured her there would be a very marked difference.

Dr Coles performs twenty surgeries a week from accident victims to a nose job, then she uses her own energy to help the patients to heal. Experiments at UCLA show that after a healing the energy surrounding the patient often begins to take on the frequency of the healer. "I feel a roughness around the area where the problem is. It causes my arm to ache a little bit" Interviewer. "So you feel the pain a little bit?" Doctor. "Yes, I keep breathing and somehow remove or exchange the negative energy".

Some want to know whether all of this would really help the patient, and we are then introduced to a lady Dr Coles had operated on and then given energy healing. She said that she could not believe that she could be so well after only three weeks since the operation. There are sceptics who say she only got well because she convinced herself she would get better. But as Dr Coles points out, she has seen the results many times and she is convinced that energy is the medicine of the future. Healing has existed in all cultures.

Even ten thousand years ago it was recorded. Healing is the one thing that has lasted throughout history. Now why would that be if it did not work?

And so we come to the end of a short but very interesting and thought provoking video. Of all the videos I have ever seen, I feel this one has to be the most enlightening and important of them all. I would not even begin to know how many times in numerous meetings and workshops around the world I have made the following statement. "I have long since learned that there is no point in saying anything unless you are someone, because no one takes any notice". When I say no one I do not mean the ordinary average citizen like the sort of people who come to those lectures or read my books. I have received endless proof over the years that those people do listen. Thousands of letters and phone calls confirm that, but when I say "no one" I am referring to the very people I need to get through to. You see Magnetic Healing is so simple in its whole concept that the highly educated, the scientist, the medical people, KNOW that nothing could be that simple and so they turn away and neither look nor listen. How true the saying, "There are none so blind as those who do not wish to see".

But the reason why I place so much importance on this tape is because, while those educated ones may not be interested in what somebody like me says or does unless they have something like professor or doctor in front of their name or several letters after it, they are quite convinced that there could be nothing of interest there for them. But when this sort of information, presented in both action pictures and voice comes from a respected surgeon with nine years of training behind her, it suddenly takes on a very different level of authenticity and importance.

There is one small comment I should make here. When Dr Coles was asked if she felt the pain she replied in the affirmative. While I cannot speak for her, I can assure you that I never feel in my body any of the pain the patient is suffering. You will recall that she had mentioned that doing the healing caused her arm to ache a little bit, and that was when she was asked if she felt the pain. Many times when I am working hard to remove a problem from a patient, my arm tenses and stiffens, and yes, I do get some pain in it, but it is nothing to do with the pain the patient has which may be in any part of her body. Any pain felt in my arm is merely created by the amount of energy flowing through it and putting it under stress, and I can only presume that this would be the sort of pain which Dr Coles would be speaking of, rather than actually taking on the pain from her patient.

And when she says that she is convinced that energy is the medicine of the future, it makes me wonder whether perhaps she has seen my fourth book. The front cover of that book shows a blown up Kirlian photo of the energy surrounding one of my sons fingers, and in the middle of it are the words, ' ENERGY, KEY OF THE FUTURE'. Strange to say, while the name of the book is actually, You Too Can Heal, I have had a number of people over the years who have either written to me or phoned me to request a copy of what they refer to as your book titled, Energy-Key of the Future. When this happens I sometimes think that surely they can see the real name of the book written in large letters across the top, so why do they use the much smaller words in the centre of the fingertip. I can only assume that there is something about this word "Energy" which stirs up within them an innate recognition of the importance of its meaning, and therefore a desire to learn more about its true significance. Hence the request for a book which they hope will give them a further insight into ways and means of using it in search of new health for their fellowman.

I think it was Nicola Tesla the inventor of alternating current and many other discoveries who said, "In that single decade when science first begins to investigate the non physical, they will make more progress in that decade than they have made in the past century." As we approach the start of a new millennium, I am filled with excitement with the thought that perhaps the first decade of that millennium may turn out to be the one which Tesla could foresee, then at long last we will finally step aside from an inhibiting so-called science, the materialistic science which has guided us down a path which can only lead to disaster for Planet Earth and its children.

Yes some doors are opening. Some scientists are beginning to recognise the need for change from low frequency physical with all its limits, to the higher frequencies, the life forces without which the physical ceases to exist. Let us then move onto another chapter, and see if we can find new and better ways of promoting their use for the benefit of mankind.

4. THE GUIDING LIGHT

Many times in my meetings I am asked the same old question, "When are we going to have the wonderful New Age of Light which people keep talking about". If that should happen to be the question on your mind, then I will give you the same answer which I have already given to thousands of people wherever I have been to speak, whether it has been in a hall, on the radio, on TV or at a small workshop where I have been showing others just how easy it is to become a channel for the Loveforce. My simple answer is always, "Never, never, never". Then I quickly add, "That is as long as you people sit back and wait for it to arrive. No Government is going to hand it to you on a plate, no religion is about to present it to you, and I do not know of any other organisation which has any intention of bringing it to you either".

The only ones I know of who can bring it about are you, and you, and you. When you can go out there and find enough courage and enough desire within yourself to spread your light and your love wide enough to encompass the greater part of the masses who are walking a path of indecision and help them to turn that turmoil in which they are enmeshed, into a path which is lighted by the fires of truth, then, and then alone will we have the New Age of light the people are seeking. It is my fervent prayer that the reading of this book will stir within its readers that courage, that desire to do their part in helping to bring it into being. You owe it, each one of you, to your children, to your children's children, and to all those who may follow in the decades to come.

But remember, if we allow the present situation to continue unabated, then some of these ones may be lucky to see the light of day at all. There must be many changes brought about for the good of mankind, and the responsibility for this rests heavily upon the shoulders of each and every individual who has been fortunate enough to have recognised this need. Do not sit back and say, "There is nothing I can do", for there is much that you can do. By spreading your light you can be an inspiration to all you meet. By the life you live you can set an example for others to follow. You can prove to many that it is not necessary for the people of Planet Earth to continue to follow this path of self destruction while the majority plod along like a flock of sheep. We are not sheep. We are individuals, each with our own distinctive set of beliefs, hopes and desires, and it is time for us to find the courage to say so. If we have a genuine desire to inspire others to follow the path of truth and to help them to raise their conscious awareness of their true soulself within and their ability to make changes for the better in their lives, then we have to begin by being a good example for them to follow.

As I approach my eightieth year in this body I look back at those years and try to see what I have done and what I have failed to do. We all make mistakes, but surely the biggest mistake of all, is to fail to learn from the ones we have already made. In this chapter I want to look back in particular at the years of my life which have passed by since I sat down to write You Too Can Heal in 1993. Perhaps together we can all learn something from my experiences during that time. Most days have been too short, and even the years seem to have raced behind me ever more quickly as each year has come and gone. There have been for me some exciting and rewarding times, but still I look back on what may have been a lost opportunity here, and a mistake there, and can only vow to try to do better in the years to come.

When my last book was first published it was not long before I began to wonder just how it had managed to be scattered so far and wide in such a short time. It all began with a phone call from Perth on the far side of Australia from New Zealand. The caller was enquiring whether it would be possible for her to come to NZ to learn to do this wonderful healing work she had been reading about in my book. It was not long before I received a couple of letters from that general area with a similar request. I decided that if there were several people wanting to travel all the way to NZ for that purpose, then it would probably be better if there was only one fare to pay. So after a few phone calls and an offer of a bed at the home of one of the very keen prospective healers, my ticket to Perth had been arranged and once again I found myself sitting back in a seat in the big bird as it lifted its wings from Auckland Airport en route to Perth.

While I had crossed the Tasman six or seven times before in this manner, I had not continued right across Australia to Perth and I looked forward to the new experiences that would await me on my arrival. I guess for most people who travel overseas, it is the scenery which they will see, the new places they will visit, plus meeting some people they have never seen before which are the big attractions. But for me it is the reverse situation. I do not go anywhere just to enjoy the scenery. That is a secondary consideration, and I look on it as a by- product of the real purpose of my journey.

The last thing I mentioned, the meeting of people I have never met before heads the list of the things which I have travelled there to do. It seems to me that many people have one big problem in their lives. They appear to have trouble getting their priorities right. For me, the purpose of my trip as always, is to reach out to as many searching souls as possible, with a view to helping them to find themselves. And when I say "Themselves" that is exactly what I mean. So many think they are the body, not being aware that what they see in the mirror is no more than the very temporary home which they have chosen to reside in for a few short years in this particular incarnation on the physical level here on Earth.

If this is the level of understanding which this one continues to hold throughout his total existence in that body from the point of time which we call birth, through to that other time which we so vaguely refer to as death, then that soul will have learnt very little in its short sojourn in the physical. But if I can help that one to gain a greater insight to his true identity as a living soul and not a mere flesh and blood human being, here today and gone tomorrow, then my flight has been well worth the effort. As you will see by the time you reach the end of this chapter, that one I have just mentioned has been multiplied many times over during my several trips to different destinations from '94 to '98.

The fourth of May '94 saw me arriving in Perth, and the fifth was a day for interviews and photographs for the newspapers, plus a 2 pm session on the University radio station. While I am not a fan for a lot of publicity, I have come to learn that no matter how keen someone may be to meet you and to learn how they can become a healer, none of this can take place if that one does not hear of your visit until after you have left. And so I have come to recognise the importance of spreading the message concerning a visit as widely as possible by whatever means is available. As I look back now through my diary for May '94, I can now see just how well that little bit of publicity worked out. Not just for me, but much more importantly, for all those who were given the opportunity of hearing what I had to say, of watching the colour slides I showed at the public meetings, and for those who attended my workshops, a chance to discover that as my previous book and my video tape tell you, you too can heal.

And how many took that opportunity when it was offered to them? Just let me do some counting here and then I can tell you. I find there were four public meetings with slides and demonstration of healing in different areas of Perth, and while I did not manage to keep a record of the numbers attending these, the teaching classes were a different story. I always tell my organisers I prefer not to have more than about twenty people attending one of these workshops as they can become too top heavy with larger numbers and each student does not have as much time to work on the patient as I would like. Looking back at those figures now I am quite amazed to find such a wide variation in numbers. Two classes were as low as nine, while by far the largest was what must have been an almost uncontrollable thirty two, a figure I would not like to repeat again.

However as there were 16 classes held during the three weeks I spent in Perth the average was near enough to 17, and a grand total of 270. A very satisfactory and rewarding visit for me, and even more so for those two hundred and seventy students. I would like to be able to tell you how many of those students who discovered their ability to heal laying dormant within them are actually continuing to use it in pursuit of new health and upliftment for their fellow beings in need. Unfortunately this information is something which I do not possess, much as I may like to. I do know that at least a few of them are because they have made the effort to contact me and to inform me of their success.

But while I find the teaching of these people to be an extremely rewarding way of using my time and energy, it can be disappointing for me to discover at some later date that many of those who put out their hands over the patient in the area I had indicated to them as being a trouble spot, have never bothered to make use of what they learnt, even though some of them were what I often refer to as a "Natural". These are the ones whose hands begin to vibrate before they have barely entered the area of the negative energy, and they start turning red as the corpuscles fill with blood.

This I find very hard to understand. It is hard for me to imagine how anyone looking at someone who is sick and perhaps suffering a lot of pain, can watch that one suffer, yet knowing that if they so desired, they could reach out their hands to their brother or sister in such need, does not bother to do so. Is it any wonder that the great founder of Homoeopathy, Samuel Hahnemann, suggested that "When we have to do with an art whose end is the saving of human life, any neglect to make ourselves masters of it becomes a crime".

I often tell a group of students that I would love to see all of them going out and healing wherever they can, but as I already know from experience, this will not happen. I have to be satisfied with the realisation that if even only one or two of them follow in my footsteps in the coming years and attend to the needs of even half of the number I have worked on through my years of healing, then my time will have been well spent.

By the time I arrived back at my home in NZ there was as usual, a pile of mail to attend to. Amongst them was a letter from Santa Fe, New Mexico, USA. Like the lady in Perth, someone had read a copy of You Too Can Heal, and wrote to check on the possibility of having me travel to US again to teach Magnetic Healing in their area. It was not long before other letters and phone calls began coming in from different areas of US, with the result that by September I was joining the birds in the air once again, but this time heading East around the planet instead of West.

I never cease to be amazed at how my friends upstairs take control at a time such as this. I mentioned in one of my previous books how a guide came through a lady in New York when I was there back in 1985. One of the interesting pieces of information he gave me was this little gem. "You do not organise the next place you will go to, the next group of people you will speak to. There is one who goes before you who does all that". And believe me this occasion in '94 was no exception.

It began with a letter from Santa Fe and finished with a grand circuit of quite a large portion of US, taking in Denver and Boulder in Colorado, across the Rockies through Vail to Glenwood Springs, on to Santa Fe, Albuquerque and Silver City in New Mexico, Bisbee in Arizona, and finally back to Los Angeles. The "One who goes before me" had done a wonderful job of organising as he always does, and to describe in any detail the whole of this journey would fill the rest of the book, but there are some highlights which I feel I must include here.

Some time before this journey began an American man who had spent most of his life in Hawaii and made a living from selling fantastic video footage of the volcanoes there, visited my home. He was at that time living with his wife in a holiday home they owned overlooking the beautiful large Lake Taupo in the centre of the North Island in NZ. He had picked up a book while walking through a bookshop in another city he had visited, and after reading it, decided he must meet the author. He explained that he had a deep desire to make some tapes of a different nature to his usual subject, and felt that he would like to begin that path with a video of the healing work which I was doing. He told me it would be a little while before he could start the work as he was going to US for a while and would be spending some time in Denver. When I enquired of him what date he expected to be there, I think he thought I was having him on when I casually mentioned that was the time I had already arranged to arrive in Denver.

And so it was after meeting me at Denver Airport, we drove across the Rockies to Glenwood Springs. A fifteen minute interview at a radio station set the tone for the rest of the journey ahead, and a well attended public meeting in a hall where my friend had set up three large professional video cameras was used as a starting point for the video of my work as a healer. The following day we held two workshops with nearly all of the participants experiencing that magic moment when they suddenly feel the Universal Energy flowing from their hands to the patient, and of course the cameras recording it for posterity.

Our next move was back across the Rockies to Boulder where the usual meetings were held, then finished up staying with one I was introduced to as Ken. He lived in a beautiful home surrounded by tree covered hills in an area known as Evergreen. It was a lovely peaceful place to spend the next three or four days with nature presenting herself in all her glory on every side. Many hours were spent working for the cameras with a patient laying on a portable couch beneath the trees, but perhaps one of the most interesting recordings we made was when Ken asked me if I could work on his large Red Setter dog which had a few problems. With Ken holding the dog's head and the cameras rolling, I placed one hand near the right leg and did not move it very far before it came up against a strong resistance to its movement.

There were a few others who were watching this operation, and they were all quite amazed to see that the moment my hand entered the area of negative energy, the dog kicked his leg away. I pulled my hand back then moved it into the area again, and each time I did this there was the same result. Surely this was a very obvious proof that even though there was no way the dog could see where my hand was, and of course it was not touching him, he was well aware that it was approaching the problem he was suffering from in that leg.

A little later my hand came along his back toward the head, and once again he tried to loosen his head from the grip of his master who was holding it as he felt the energy from my hand interacting with the negative energy in that area. Ken could not get over the fact that while he had not told me anything about the problems with his dog, he knew that the right leg and the head were the two areas where he was having trouble. Sometimes when I work on a dog in this way, he will not only try to move the offending part of his body away from my hand as it approaches, but will set up a deep growling, and on a few occasions have actually made a little snap at my hand at the precise moment that I break something away from his body. I never get the impression that the dog is actually trying to bite my hand, but it is his way of saying, "I felt that".

I feel that all of this is a very important and positive piece of evidence for the proof of the interaction of fields between the healer and the one being healed. Surely if as medical people have told me many times, "You can't possibly do anything by just moving your hands over a body" or "The patient is only imagining they feel something because they want to", then how do we explain the reaction of animals in this way. Do they growl at me or take a little snap at my hand only in the very moment that I actually draw something away from their bodies because they imagine they feel something happening?

There are times when some doctor or scientist refuses to accept that anything at all is really happening when I run my hands through the energy field of a patient, when I am tempted to say something like, "The dogs must know more about it than you do". But at least as we saw in chapter three, doors are beginning to open, and now at last, after thirty years of attempting to break through that barrier which these people have surrounded themselves with for so long, I feel a surge of elation beginning to fill my very being as one after another these barriers begin to crumble and I become ever more aware that those years of effort have not been wasted.

Back in US my next flight was to Albuquerque and on to Santa Fe. One full week in this very interesting place was filled with radio broadcasts, public meetings and workshops, and many a budding healer was left behind me when I was finally taken back to Albuquerque to spend a few days there. A late night interview on a radio station brought an unexpected response. The next morning there was a call from a well known anchorman at KRQETV. He rang to say he had been listening to the radio the previous evening and was fascinated by what he had heard me saying. He wanted to know if I would be a part of his midday show tomorrow. I agreed to do so but was amazed to find that this time I would not be going to a studio but would be interviewed on a street at the New Mexico State Fair which happened to be running that week.

The lady I was staying with drove me out to this amazing place with acres of streets and buildings like a small town. No cars were allowed in, but we followed our TV man in his car and he informed the guards that the car behind him was a part of his show today, and we drove through after a sticker had been placed on our windscreen. Thousands of people milled around from street to street and building to building and for someone who had come from a little town containing three thousand five hundred people on the other side of the world I may as well have been on Mars, such was the contrast to anything I could ever be likely to see at home.

At the corner of one street stood a large van with aerials protruding from it and several workers with earphones and other equipment preparing for the show. This began with our anchorman, Ted, reading the news in front of cameras set up in the street with picture and sound going to the van from where it was sent to the main transmitter in the city and directly to the viewers. After the news, while I stood to one side anxiously waiting my turn, he interviewed the wife of the mayor of Albuquerque, and I am thinking that at least I am in good company. As she moved away at the end of her interview, I was motioned to move forward as the cameras rolled, and Ted began to question me concerning the healing work I had been doing for so long.

It was good to know that out there were thousands of viewers in that big city and its environs who were hearing first hand, some of them possibly for the first time what you can do to heal the sick by allowing yourself to be used as a channel for the Loveforce. Call it Universal energy, call it Godforce if you wish. Names do not change it. It is, and it is everywhere, and it is free. No hidden costs for this drug or that potion, and no nasty side effects which so many of these can bring about in an unsuspecting patient. After the interview was over, Ted's Midday Show concluded and they packed up their gear and returned to the city. As we had a sticker of identification on our window we reckoned we may as well stay for a while, have something to eat at one of the many food distributing areas and have a look around. While we were doing this we had a very interesting discussion with a government man at one of the stalls, but I would prefer to leave that incident to be included in a later chapter where I will be discussing other aspects of the many uses of energy.

The next three days were busy ones with the usual roundup of public meetings and workshops, one of which was attended by Ted and his wife. Monday morning saw me sitting in a twenty seater Beechcraft 1900 with just three other passengers on our way to Silver City. The area around this city tends to be very hilly so the Airport is about twenty miles out in the country on the nearest piece of flat land large enough to build one on. A public meeting and a workshop were held on consecutive days at the University, with a second class the last day at the home where I was staying.

The following morning my bags were placed in a car belonging to a friend of the lady I had been staying with, and we set off for Bisbee in Arizona. On the way we called in to see the Tyrone copper mine. And what an exciting two and a half hours we spent there. An eight seater air-conditioned mini bus was laid on for us free of charge, and we were driven on a circuitous route through every part of the mine. Then came another three hour drive to Bisbee. Of all the many places I have had the pleasure of visiting around the world, the little town of Bisbee will always hold a tender spot in my memory. There are several reasons for this. For a start, Waihi where I live in NZ is a small goldmining town. The underground mine which was responsible for the creation of the town back around 1878, was finally closed in 1952, but has since been opened again, this time as an open cast mine with the result that what used to be known as Martha Hill has now become Martha Hole as the hill was gradually removed in order to claim the gold which had been left by the underground method,

When I was driven into Bisbee, here was a quaint little town with an old underground mine and an open cast one. Admittedly they had been copper mines and not gold, but the thing that struck me most was the fact that this was the only other place I had been to where there was a mine virtually at the end of the main street, I immediately felt at home, because Waihi is exactly like that. But very soon there were other good reasons for feeling at home. The people who had invited me here had once been to my home in NZ when they were living in my country for a while. They were well into the understanding of energy and its uses, were authors of a book titled "The I Ching Made Easy" and had a programme on a local radio station. As well as the home they lived in, they owned another house where I stayed for the week I spent in Bisbee. This house had quite a large room where they held meetings, so this meant we could hold all of our workshops right there, and when it was finished, if it was an evening one I could go straight to bed without having to travel anywhere.

The first day in Bisbee Rod and Amy drove me to Sierra Vista, a town of about eight thousand people where we did another radio interview. Saturday evening was public meeting night. The hall was privately owned, and John the owner, told me his donation would be free use of the hall for the evening. This must have been one of the few places I had ever held a public meeting without having to pay for the hire of the hall. Wherever I go and whatever I do, be it a public meeting, a workshop or a healing, for all of these I rely on the generosity of the people to cover my costs of hall hire, any advertising and my travel. My wife and I have lived very well for the past twenty five years on the proceeds of a donation box and continue to do so.

But here in Bisbee, if I felt good about the generosity of John in offering to give me his hall for free for the evening, I was even more elated as the people came through the door to take their seats in the hall. There was something about these people which I could not quite put my finger on. They seemed to be filled with a desire to learn whatever I may be able to teach them, and it was not very early that night by the time the last of them asked their final question and we were able to lock up and go home to bed. I knew that here in Bisbee there would be some wonderful workshops to follow that public meeting.

And I was not wrong. Four classes over the next two days saw almost eighty very keen students try their hand at feeling the negative energy on the volunteer patients, and the great majority of them went away with a smile of satisfaction on their faces at the prospect of now being able to help their friends when they are sick. One day of rest before my good friends Rod and Amy drove me through the well known little town of Tombstone, and on to Tucson where I boarded a plane for Los Angeles. But just before we leave that lovely little town of Bisbee behind us, there is one more very important mention of it I need to make. In front of me at this moment I have a very small yellow piece of paper with some writing on it. A while ago I received a book from Rod and Amy and sticking to it was this piece of paper.

It didn't look very important, but the short message they had written on it was the best piece of news I had received in some time. It simply said, "Dear Colin, You will be pleased to know that several healing groups are continuing your good work. Best wishes, Rod and Amy". Pleased they said. That was an understatement. I was elated. Now I knew for sure that what I had expected to take place there really had eventuated. Another lamp had been lit during my visit, and now in my absence it continued to burn brightly for all to see.

I was met at LA Airport by Suzanne who drove me to the lovely home in Altadena which she shared with her husband Tim, a computer equipment manufacturer. They had a very large lounge and we had forty two people there the following evening to see my slides and a demonstration of Magnetic Healing. Two classes were held there, eighteen in the first and twenty two in the second. I see by my notes that by the time we came to the end of that one there had been a total of three hundred and seventeen students who had attended the workshops on that little jaunt around a portion of US, and I feel that my effort made to spread the light of understanding in those areas was well rewarded.

But more, much more was to follow between the trip to US and this present time of writing. One of the questions people keep asking me is when I am going to retire. They say that most people at seventy nine are sitting back and enjoying their twilight years. I tell them I may not be sitting back but I am enjoying life like I have never enjoyed it before. When you realise that you are using each day granted to you to do that which you came onto the Earthplane in this incarnation to do, then your inner joy and satisfaction knows no bounds. Why would I want to sit back and wait to die when I know it would not take long for that to happen if I was foolish enough to fill my mind with such negative thoughts. That sort of thinking pattern is for the elderly. I simply tell them I am sorry, but I do not have time to think about that. I have too much to do to occupy my mind and body for as long as permission is given to me to do so. As long as there are dark corners anywhere, then I know it is my duty to attempt to light a candle in that place to help to disperse some of the dark shadows of ignorance which many still live under as they struggle their way through life.

In January '96 as I opened a letter with a Vancouver, Canada postmark, I wondered who could be writing to me as Canada was a country I had not yet visited. The letter it contained was from a man who had not long retired from school teaching and had visited a doctor only to be told that he was suffering from a very serious cancer and had only a matter of months to live. Naturally he and his family were shattered by the news and began to make plans for the inevitable.

A short time after this his daughter came home from visiting a bookshop in the city, and in her hand was a copy of "You Too Can Heal". I had no idea any copies had reached Canada at all, but apparently like Perth and Santa Fe they were available in bookshops there. She handed it to her father and after reading it, and sensing a little glimmer of hope he wrote to me to ask me if I would consider giving him some absent healing. I will be writing a chapter in this book titled "Absent Healing" for those who may not understand exactly what is meant by that expression, so do not despair at this stage if you are not familiar with this method of healing, as I can assure you all will be revealed before my pen is finally laid aside.

When I had read this letter, I tucked it under a button at the lower end of my healing couch. I then placed the fingers of my right hand on the signature at the bottom of the letter and mentally asked for that one whose name I was now seeing in my minds eye to be placed on the couch in front of me. As always, I said to myself, "We will now work to clear the blood of this body", and as I did so I placed my right hand in the area where I knew his left foot would have been if he had been there in the physical form. As I moved my hand slowly up the couch, visualising the artery beneath it, a lot of pressure began to build up in front of it, and it was not long before I found it very difficult to move my hand forward at all.

After spending some time and energy clearing the blood from foot to heart on both legs, my hand approached the torso and I asked to be shown where the source of this problem could be found. It was not long before my hand came up against what I sometimes refer to as a brick wall and more time was spent drawing this energy away and discarding it well away from my couch. A few days later I decided to check the body again, and was pleased to find that although there was still some negative energy to be removed the pressure my hand came up against was considerably less, and not nearly as much time was spent in order to clear the area so that my hand would run freely over the whole length of the couch without coming up against any resistance.

After repeating this procedure another two or three times over the next week or two, just to make sure there was nothing more to be found in his energy field, I wrote to him in Vancouver, and it was not long before I received a phone call from him, telling me how much better he was feeling. This all took place in January of '96, but by March I had received another letter from my patient and his wife. They were writing to say that owing to the miracle of healing which had taken place in his body, they would like to send me Airline return tickets to Vancouver and have me stay at their home as their guest for two or three weeks. This caused something of a dilemma for me. My life is a busy one, and I have a purpose in that life. I could not imagine putting aside that purpose just to go holidaying when I could have spent that precious time helping those in need of healing.

Then it suddenly occurred to me that I should be able to combine the two, doing some healing, and maybe even better still, showing some people in Vancouver how they could become better healers. My friend had written his phone number in his letter, so I pushed a few buttons and very soon found myself talking to my patient. He sounded like he was just a little taken aback when I suggested that if he would organise a public meeting in a hall and perhaps some teaching classes then I would be very happy to take up his offer. However, he requested some assistance from his sister who lived about twenty miles to the South and between them they did a wonderful job of organising not one, but four public meetings in different areas, including one in the St Johns United Church in Sechelt, and another in the Church of Truth in Victoria the Capital of British Columbia on Vancouver Island.

But even more importantly they had several workshops organised for me where I could teach my method of healing to a large number of very keen students. As always this number was continuously added to, because at the end of a public meeting we always ask for a show of hands of those who would like to become healers, and usually we finish up with at least one or two more classes organised before the meeting comes to a close.

In one of my previous books I have mentioned how I was fortunate to have a Kirlian machine built for me by the husband of a lady who came to me for healing several times from a city about forty miles from my home. She was suffering from a very rare disease and the doctor had given her a few months at the most at the time she first came to me. But owing to the healing I was able to give her, those few months were extended to around what her husband often referred to later as six wonderful years. About half way through that time he offered to build me a Kirlian machine to enable me to take pictures of the energy field around the fingers such as the one you see on page 121.

These people spent most of their life in Canada and had only come to live in NZ after retirement. After the wife finally passed on the husband decided to return to Canada and I lost all track of him. But while staying with my friends in Vancouver, I had a feeling that I had heard him mention that city a few times when he had brought his wife to me for healing, and decided to take a look through the telephone book just in case this happened to be the city he had returned to. Of course I was not even aware whether he would still be alive as he was getting on a bit by the time he left to return to Canada. We did find a name which looked as if it may belong to him as it had the correct initial for his Christian name. We had a little trouble getting through to him as he had not long shifted to a different house and his number had been changed. When I did finally reach him and gave him my name and informed him I was in Vancouver, he sounded as if he could hardly believe what he was hearing.

Since he made that Kirlian machine for me I have taken many photos with it, some of which I have had made into slides. These have been shown to hundreds of people in gatherings in the several countries I have had the pleasure and privilege of visiting, and so many have for the first time been given positive proof that every living thing has this lifeforce flowing through it and surrounding it. From experience I am well aware that just seeing this energy shown on the screen, and of course in my books as well, has changed the whole belief and understanding of many of them.

With this in mind I decided to set up a projector with some slides in it showing some of the photos on the day that he said he would visit us. When we saw him arriving at the house, I switched on the projector so that it showed a very large fingertip with a beautiful aura of energy pouring from it on the wall of the lounge. We opened the door and he and I greeted each other like the long lost friends that we were. I then stood back and waited as he walked further into the room. He did not go very far before he noticed this strange looking picture covering a large part of one wall. He looked really puzzled and then enquired as to what he was actually looking at. I simply said, "You did that", he was obviously still at a loss to understand what I meant, so I pushed the button a few times on the projector and several different photos of the energy fields followed one after another on the wall.

I explained how his making of that Kirlian machine several years ago had done so much in different areas to change the thinking pattern of so many people. When the last one finally gave way to a blank wall as I pushed the button for the last time, I stood back and waited for his response. It was slow in coming, but when it did I thought I could detect a little moisture in the corner of my eye as this grand old man, now in his eighties, said very slowly, "Well Colin, it looks as if I did something useful with my life after all". Tears were already showing in his eyes, and I felt that he was thinking about all those years, probably back to the day when he stood at the door of my home now so far away in NZ and proudly handed me the completed machine. And I was remembering that day too. I was remembering how I could hardly believe that I actually had in my hand a Kirlian machine of my own, when at that time there would have been very few if any in the country.

I could also remember how, after carrying it into the healing room I asked him how much I owed him for all the parts he had bought for it and his work. He looked at me as if I had said something which hurt him. Then in a voice I had never quite heard before, he said, "Please don't insult me. Do you really think that after all you have done to give Molly and me these extra years together which we were not supposed to have, I could charge you for this?"

As we stood there in that lovely home so far away in both time and distance, I felt that by showing him those photos and allowing him to see something of the results of his work, I had at long last in a roundabout way been able to offer him something in return for his efforts. All is not lost on Planet Earth. There are still some very good simple people out there who know the meaning of love, and who are aware that if they can spend their days spreading a little of their light and their love for their fellow beings ever more widely, then the greed and the lust for power can be swept away and the time we refer to as the New Age can be ushered in in all its glory. But do not leave it for your neighbour to do, because he is probably doing the same, and two negatives can never make a positive. Nature does not work that way, and neither can we.

Some of my readers may be disappointed when I tell you that about a year after I worked on my Vancouver friend he suddenly became very ill and passed away. Perhaps you are asking yourself whether there was any point in giving him the healing in the first place, so let me explain to you how I see this series of events as I look back on it now. If his daughter had not bought a copy of my book and taken it home to him, he would never have known there was any alternative to the previous path he had been following. He would have simply done what most people do. He would have accepted the doctor's findings and believed there was nothing to be done which could give him even a few extra months of good life. He would have expected to pass on within the short time the doctor had predicted, and I have no doubt he would have done so, judging by the condition he was in the first time I worked on him.

It was good that he was given those extra months with his family, and it was great that he was able to have me in his home and to spend the third week of my visit there driving me and his wife on a long sightseeing journey up into the Rocky Mountains. But all this really fades into insignificance when you take a good look at the real reason why that book came into the hands of his daughter as she walked through the bookshop. If it had not, then I would never have made the trip to Canada. You see, I have long since come to learn that these things do not come about by accident. If you work with Spirit, they work with you. As the guide in New York had said, "You do not plan the next place you will go to, the next group of people you will speak to. There is one who goes before you who does all that".

Yes, how true. And it had to start with a man who was virtually dying of cancer. There were two separate paths which could have been followed here. Spirit could have said, "Well, his time on Earth is due to come to an end for this incarnation, so we will let him follow that path and he can come over and join us very soon". But there was a possible alternative to that, and I believe that is the one they took. By looking at this alternative path they could see that everybody could gain a great deal by allowing him to follow it. It was a simple matter of making sure his daughter was guided to pick up a particular book and take it home for her father to read.

They would know that once this path had been shown to him he would follow it even though he would at that time have no idea whatsoever where it would lead. Oh yes, of course he would be hoping that by following it he would gain a little extra time with his wife and family, and important as that may have been to him I am sure that in the long term plan which Spirit would have seen from their perspective, that would have been a very small portion of the extent of the overall plan as it was to unfold. If the book had never been delivered into his hands, there would have been today a lot more sick people in the Vancouver area. It is true that while I was there I was able to heal a very limited number of people, but it must be realised that since that time many more have gained new health, and for a lot of them, a whole new understanding of life.

There were those who came to my public meetings. They saw the slides. They heard me spending two hours explaining what they were all about. They watched me through the third hour doing a demonstration of Magnetic Healing on a patient. But there were also those who owing to their desire to be of service to their fellow beings made the extra effort to attend a workshop so that they could discover within themselves their latent ability to heal. And many did exactly this. As always there were those who broke down in tears as they found their hands pulsing with energy and lifting the negativity away from ailing bodies for the first time in their lives.

None of this would have taken place if it had not been for the message in that book finding its way into the hands and the heart of the cancer sufferer. It is my humble prayer that this collection of words I am sitting here bringing together to form what we refer to as a book, will be used to continue the work of spreading the light in whatever form they wish to use it.

And how do I know just how much light was spread in that area in the short time I spent there? Well, for me, perhaps the most rewarding moment in connection with the whole plan as it unfolded, actually took place in my home a few months later. The phone rang, and I picked it up to hear a female voice asking me if she was speaking to Mr Lambert the healer. I assured her she was, and she went on to say that she was ringing me from Vancouver. She said there were three other ladies standing beside her and they had all been students at one or other of the classes I had held there some time ago. She went on to say that they had decided to get together to ring me up and say thank you for coming to Vancouver and changing our lives. I was just thinking how wonderful it was to be given a message like that from the other side of the world, when she added something even more significant. She said, "not only our lives, but the lives of all those people we are now giving healing to".

What a wonderful moment. The plan had been fulfilled in its entirety, yet it would actually never end. This was only four I had heard from, but I knew there would be many more I knew nothing of who were continuing to spread the light, each in their own way. Extracts from two of the letters I have received from Vancouver also show how the flame of truth can light the way for those whose minds are open enough to seek it. "Dear Colin, I am writing to thank you for travelling to Canada with your healing message and your healing touch, I admire your enthusiasm and insight. I believe the earth is in a period of profound transformation, and this is reflected in the change that so many people are experiencing in their lives at this time. Health problems are very much a part of this transformation".

And from another, "Meeting you has been a heavenly experience, You have profoundly changed my life. Words cannot describe the changes that have taken place in the way I feel physically, mentally and Spiritually. You are a wonderful person. (Just a very simple ordinary guy as far as I am concerned.) and a great teacher. Your message is simple and direct, but unfortunately our minds (computers) have been programmed otherwise, and it is a matter of reprogramming and going back to basics. Cancer has been an awakening call for me, and thank you for contributing to that awakening. Good luck in your mission. You have succeeded in planting seeds which will blossom into beautiful flowers. Love and respect. M."

And so the torch of truth is carried like an Olympic flame from one to another, forever gaining in strength and brightness, never to be extinguished as long as enough of you can find the courage, the desire, and the determination to keep it burning. The truth will set you free. Step into the light and bathe in the glory of its warmth.

5. FEEDBACK

1997 was a year for staying in NZ and travelling to numerous different areas which included several public meetings, and according to my diary at least thirty workshops. There was a visit to England amongst all that, but for a very good reason it is my intention to leave that to be part of chapter six. Towards the latter end of the year "The one who goes before me and does all that" began to show some very positive signs of moving me in the direction of another trip to Australia. I had some friends I had stayed with in Melbourne on a previous visit, who had written to me to ask me when I was going to return to Australia. They had by this time shifted to a small town by the name of Milton about two hundred Kilometres south of Sydney. I had promised them I would visit them in their new locality when the opportunity arose but could give them no date at that time. My flight to England had left me with enough Air Points to cover a free return flight to Australia, but I did not want to use them for that purpose unless there was a chance of making the best possible use of them by visiting other areas to lecture and to teach.

While contemplating this possibility, I received a phone call from Auckland. A man and his wife from Tasmania were spending a few days in the city and had seen a copy of the You Too Can Heal book and were very keen to travel down to Waihi to visit me. They did so the following day, and apart from giving them some healing we had a long discussion concerning our various beliefs and understandings, mostly of a Spiritual nature. Before they left they questioned me as to the possibility of visiting them at their home in Tasmania sometime. They assured me they would not only be delighted to have me stay with them, but would be honoured to be given the opportunity of organising public meetings and workshops in Tasmania following the pattern of those which I had been telling them I had been doing in NZ and other countries. I told them how I had been considering a visit to my friends in Milton, and suggested there could be a good chance of fitting in a visit to Tasmania at the same time. I had them write out their names, address and phone number so that I would be able to contact them if and when I decided to go there.

Barely a week went by before I found myself answering the phone again under very similar circumstances. Once again it was from some people who were passing through NZ and had stopped in Auckland for a few days. They had heard of my work as a healer from someone they had been speaking to in Auckland, and as the husband was not a very well man, decided to ring me to see if they could have an appointment for some healing. And yes, you guessed it. Just like the other two, they came down to my home, had some healing, talked a lot, then asked me if there was any possibility that I may be visiting Australia to lecture and teach in the near future. They told me they had a lovely home in Melbourne and would be delighted to have me stay with them. As they already knew quite a few people who were into this type of work in Melbourne, they felt they would have no problem organising meetings etc.

This time, my response was just a little different. I found it difficult not to have a broad smile on my face as I said, "OK You win". They probably wondered what I was talking about, and could not have known that rather than saying those words to them, I was really speaking to the one who goes before me to arrange all that. I felt that the time had arrived for me to recognise that all this was a little more than could be sensibly labelled "coincidence" so my answer to them in this case contained more of the affirmative than the one I gave to my visitors the previous week. Again I made sure they left me all the relevant details and assured them I would be in contact with them in the near future.

The plan my friend upstairs appeared to be formulating for me seemed to be falling into place very nicely. Any reader who knows anything about the topography of the Continent of Australia will be aware that the Island of Tasmania is situated off the extreme south of the mainland, while Melbourne is the first large city to be encountered flying north, and my friends in Milton were about another two hundred miles further north. By starting my journey from Tasmania and continuing northward from there, I could then go on to Sydney and fly home from there. But I suppose I should have known that it would not be quite as simple as that.

This was confirmed a few days later when a letter arrived from Brisbane, further north still, with a similar request to the others. A home to stay in, meetings to be arranged, transport provided etc. This had to be it. Now there could be no doubts. All of this was obviously something they wished me to do, and I knew that this would not be happening unless someone up there was well aware that many people in those areas had reached the stage where they were seeking the eternal truths and were just waiting for someone to come along and show them the path which they would need to follow. Long before I came to the end of that trip and was ready to wing my way back across the Tasman sea, I knew that I had not been wrong in that respect.

Plans came together almost effortlessly, and by the end of February '98 I was looking down at Launceston, a city in the more northern part of Tasmania. Penny and Jerome who had visited my home a few months earlier were there to meet me but as they lived some distance from Launceston we stayed at a motel there for the next two nights. I had travelled from my home that morning, a two-hour drive to Auckland Airport, a long flight to Melbourne, and a change of planes for a shorter flight to Launceston. The day was dragging on by the time I finally arrived there, and I was just thinking my bed at the motel would be a very welcome place quite early this evening when they dropped the bomb.

They casually mentioned that everything was arranged for this evening's public meeting. Oh no! Travelling all day and now standing for three hours showing slides, continuously talking to explain to the audience what they were all about, and doing a demonstration of Magnetic Healing on a patient. All this on top of my long flight. I remember thinking it was just as well my body was a very young seventy-eight.

However, as usual it all went off like clock work, and it was obvious the audience enjoyed the evening with many of them asking to be included in the workshop the following day. Sunday we drove to the south of Tasmania where we were booked into a large hotel for a couple of days. That evening our meeting was held in a large room at the hotel, and my notes for that night are brief and to the point. "Sixty people. Excellent meeting". I always find that the number of people coming to a meeting is very much an unknown quantity. Just when you think there will be a good attendance at a particular meeting, they let you down and the number can be disappointingly small, but on another occasion when you are not expecting many to arrive, perhaps because you feel the meeting has not been well advertised, that is just the time they surprise you by turning up in droves.

We had arranged for two workshops the following day, one in the morning and another in the afternoon. I always try to have the organisers arrange two meetings like this so that roughly an equal number attend each class as I do not like to have more than twenty to teach at a time. There was a total of forty-two who came to the classes that day, and around twenty or so at each meeting would have been great. I must admit it was a little disappointing to see only twelve students arrive for the morning class, and decided that there could not have been as many keen prospective healers at last nights public meeting as I thought. But as I waited for everyone to settle down at the afternoon meeting so that I could get started, I began to think they were not going to stop coming through the door.

And they didn't until more than thirty very keen looking students were sitting in front of me anxiously awaiting the start of the class. Oh well, you win some, and you lose some. But judging by the comment I made in my notes concerning this class, we certainly didn't lose this one in spite of the overload. The two words "Terrific meeting " said it all. While I have not had any official information concerning how many of these are continuing to be used as channels for the healing energy, I am sure that from what I remember of some of those who stepped up to the couch and discovered they were one of those I refer to as a "natural", there will be at least some of them who are doing so. I have said many times, and I will say it again, if just one of those who attend a class goes out and continues to use what they have learnt over the following years, then my time and energy will have been well spent.

My visit to Melbourne on my first leg north was in some respects a strange one, mainly for the fact that what I have just said about losing one and gaining one, and not knowing how many will turn up to a meeting was born out more fully than in any other place I have visited. At the public meeting on the Saturday evening there were seven members of the family I was staying with who came to the hall, and would you believe there were just three members of the public. I could not understand what went wrong then, and I still don't, particularly in view of the fact that when we held a workshop two days later I was saddled with another one of those crazy thirty people classes. I can only imagine that the few who did attend the public meeting must have gone around telling their friends what they had missed, so they decided to catch up on it by coming to the workshop.

An all night bus trip from Melbourne saw me in Milton early next morning where my friends awaited my arrival. That evening we held a small but very good meeting at Ron and Diane's home, and the following evening they drove me to their friends home at Nowra where an excellent class of twenty three people showed a very keen interest in learning to become healers. The best way I can report the results of this meeting is to quote from a card which was sent to me a few months later.

"Dear Colin, Since your healing visit to Australia in March this year, Helen and I have had several healing sessions at our north Nowra home. Photographic evidence of a May session is enclosed as proof of your spreading your Spiritual work worldwide. (Photo page 121). Spirit is no doubt pleased with your efforts, and we indeed thank you for being as you are. Thank you for all that you have done. (Barry.)"

I suppose you could say, well, that says it all, but another letter from Milton adds another chapter to the mounting evidence which must surely finally prove to a sceptical "Scientific" fraternity that there really is more, much more, out there to be understood than just that low frequency physical level with all its limiting factors. A level which they appear to be determined to cling to, afraid that to open their minds to any alternative would suddenly sweep from beneath them all the time and effort they have spent learning about that level.

"Dear Colin, I am writing to thank you for coming over in March to Milton and showing us your way of Magnetic Healing. At the time I was sceptical and overwhelmed, and now even more so as I am now doing the work myself which I feel very privileged to be doing. So a sincere and very big thank you for making such a difference in not only my life, but a lot of other peoples lives. You are a very special person".

Before I make any other comments here, I feel I must once again address that last sentence. So often a writer puts something like this in their correspondence to me, and I want to point out to you that whatever they may think I do not believe that statement is necessarily a true one. I suppose, in their eyes this is how they see me, simply because I come into their midst, and a bit like a whirlwind, I stir up the dust and totally change the scene. Just as the dust and a lot of useless debris can be swept away by that wind, so a lot of old beliefs and useless baggage is suddenly swept aside when someone opens the door marked "TRUTH", and the light of that truth floods in.

I well remember one lady who rang me to congratulate me on my last book. She began by saying, "Mr Lambert, I am half way through your wonderful book". After letting her rattle on for a while about what she thought of it, I finally stopped her and asked her if she could just answer one question for me. She wanted to know what that question was, so I put it to her. I asked her why it was that she, like a lady from a very different part of

NZ that very morning, plus several others at different times, have either phoned me or written to me to tell me as she had done, that they were half way through my book. Why had they not waited until they had finished it before contacting me?

There was quite a long silence on the phone and I felt I could almost hear the wheels going round as she contemplated the answer she would give me. Then slowly it came. Slowly and directly as she said, "I can't answer for the other people, but for me, I think it is just that on every page there seems to be something which says inside of me, I knew that, I have always known that, but I have never had the courage to say so to anyone in case they thought I was strange. But now I have found someone with enough courage to put it down on paper for all of us to read. That is why I just had to ring you and thank you".

That answer was so typical of many statements in my mail or my phone calls. And perhaps it is because at last they have found someone, as she put it, with enough courage to put it down on paper for all to see. But I do not see how that makes me anything special. It does mean I am not afraid to face the truth, as many appear to be. For me, there is only one thing worth giving any consideration, and that is truth. I often tell people that if there is any difference between me and them, then maybe it is just my total recognition of what I really am. Perhaps you have not come to the realisation of your true soulself within. Maybe you do not know that the physical body which you are residing in at this time is no more than the overcoat which you have put on and will wear for as long as you are here in that physical form on the earthplane in order to learn lessons which you could not learn without that physical body to work through.

For me it is that total recognition which brings with it the acceptance of your oneness with all that is. The understanding that you cannot raise your hand in anger against your brother without hurting yourself because you are all one. It is because I know that we can never have that wonderful New Age of Light until the living souls of this planet arrive at that level of understanding, that I have put so much time and effort into trying to do my part in spreading this simple truth.

It was just a few months ago that I was running a workshop in the South Island, when a young man I would guess to be in his late teens came up to me and spoke to me in what I suppose one would have to describe as modern day language, but hardly the word we would have used when I was his age. He simply said, "Mr Lambert, I have never met anyone like you. You are awesome". I could not help smiling a little at his way of expressing his feelings towards me, but I knew it was telling me a great deal. I knew that something I had said or done during that meeting had hit the spot I had been aiming at. It told me that here was a young man with a whole life ahead of him, who had suddenly discovered there was a new and very different path for him to follow through that life, and I knew that from this moment on his life would never be quite the same.

I could see that now he would no longer blindly accept everything the powers that be told him he should take on board without even giving it a second thought as to whether it really was the truth or not. At last he would begin to use what his creator had given him to think with. I have long since come to realise that this is something which the great majority of people rarely do. They listen to a scientist a minister of religion, or maybe if they are naive enough, even a politician, and they say to themselves, he is the expert on these matters, he must know.

But don't you believe it. Truth is the last thing they will tell you, simply because they know that if you find it they will lose you. Religion lost me quite a few years ago when I discovered that the story they had told me in my Baptist Church and Sunday School about being a naughty sinner the day I was born and so I should be kneeling to Him out there somewhere and asking for forgiveness did not fit in with the very positive statements I found in the Bible one day. "The Kingdom of God is within you".

So He was not out there somewhere after all. He was right here within me and within you. I could see the people picking up stones to stone Him at a time when He had incarnated in the flesh in order to be able to bring once again His wonderful message of love to His brothers and sisters of Planet Earth. I could hear Him asking them why they would want to stone him, and I could hear them telling Him that it was because He dared to call Himself God and could not allow Him to blaspheme their creator in this way. But most of all, I felt I could hear Him replying to them with these words "IS IT NOT WRITTEN IN YOUR LAW, I HAVE SAID, YE ARE GODS."

For those of you who read my last book I make no excuses for having written this before. For you it will serve as a reminder, and for those who have not read it, then maybe it will bring to your notice something which you were not yet aware of. A small group of words which I often refer to as the three most important words in the Bible. (St John. 10—34) You may notice that verse 38 ends in this way. "The Father is in me, and I in Him" Surely then in telling us that like Him, we are gods, then is he not also saying the father is in you and you in Him? What a tragedy it has been for mankind that organised religion throughout the ages has failed to recognise the truth of His simple statements, and in so doing has held the people in bonds of fear and persecution.

But of course all of this is no more than a conceived plan to keep the simple truth from the masses. They are well aware that if they were to discover this, then they would want their freedom and the hold over them would be broken. They know that the truth is the one thing which will set them free. Free to think for themselves. At long last free to understand that they do not need a priest or minister to intercede for them. Free to know that they only need to seek within themselves where that divine spark of God lies, waiting for you to recognise the soulself which is the real you. Soul incarnate, soul discarnate. Incarnate within the physical for a few short years, or discarnate in that other form from whence you came at birth and will return when your short sojourn in the physical form ceases. Incarnate or discarnate, you are still a divine spark of all that is.

You may have noticed that both of the letters quoted from mention the changes which have taken place since I visited the area. One of them tells of the resultant bringing together of like-minded people to work on each other or to give healing to anyone who needs it, while the other is on a more personal level. She is reporting to me something of the changes which have taken place in her life. From a sceptic being overwhelmed by what she felt as her hands entered the negative area in the patient's aura, to the joy she now feels each time she reaches out her hands to one who comes to her for assistance with a health problem. Hence the name of this chapter, "Feedback". For that is what it is, and if I was to copy in this book all the many similar letters, or put on paper the similar expressions of gratitude which have been relayed to me by telephone, I would have little room for anything else. Such is the response which comes back to me from those who I have had the pleasure and privilege of being able to help to discover within themselves their latent ability to be used as channels for the energy of the universe.

When my work was finished in the Milton – Nowra area, my friends drove me to Sydney where I stepped onto a plane bound for Brisbane where a whole new round of exciting events was to take place. The strange thing about all this is the fact that while I do almost the identical work of lecturing and teaching at each place I visit, there are never two places the same. This begins with the people I stay with. They are all different. They have different levels of understanding. They have formulated long before I arrive, a plan which they hope will bring into their area the maximum benefit from my visit for as many people as possible. Nine times out of ten this works out very well and Brisbane was certainly no exception. Yet in spite of all the efforts of my organisers we found ourselves with slide projector ready and the clock already sliding past start time, and an unbelievable fifteen people sitting in a large hall at the University.

Just why this happens still remains a mystery to me, but there is one thing I have noticed, and this applies not only to NZ but in most countries I visit. I know it may sound silly, but all too many times I have found that the larger the city, the smaller the number of people in the hall. As we saw with Melbourne, so it was with Brisbane. There have been a few cities where a large number have attended, but that is the exception rather than the norm. I have given quite a lot of thought to this, and tried to figure out why this should be. Surely one would expect that the greater the number of people living within a short distance of the hall where the meeting is taking place, the larger the audience will be. Why then does it not work out that way? After many years of travelling I have come up with a few conclusions about this strange phenomenon, so I place them here for your consideration.

Firstly there can be the odd occasion where my organisers have not done as good a job as they thought they had, but I am sure this would only account for a very small amount of the cities where the people fail to turn up. So there has to be other reasons. I think at this time of little Bisbee in Arizona, a small isolated town which I have already mentioned, and once again I see a happy smiling crowd of obviously interested people coming into the hall looking as if they were really expecting an enjoyable and instructive evening. Then I see the time when the meeting had just come to a close, and still hear the sound of the spontaneous clapping. It was as if they were saying they had come with expectations which for them had been fulfilled in their entirety. And always in these smaller towns I find myself surrounded with those who are keen to learn a little more, and they gather around to ask questions or to listen to the answers I am giving to those who have asked. I always feel at this time that I am among friends, yet these are people that I have never met before.

At this stage I can only hope that my city dwelling readers will not be offended when I tell them this rarely happens in quite the same way or to the same degree when I lecture in larger cities. But I can only report here what I have found to be true over many years. So perhaps it is time for us to give some thought as to why this should be so. Should there be any difference between the city dweller and his cousin in the small town forty or fifty miles away? And if there is then why is it so. Perhaps we could surmise that in the city there are many very different ways of spending your leisure time, and so people tend to attend some function which they feel is most important to them. It may be a movie, a dance, or a hotel bar or one of the numerous ways of entertainment which are available in a large city.

But in a small town, not a lot happens. In our little town of about three and a half thousand people for instance, we no longer have a movie theatre, so most of those who want to see a movie, either watch one on TV or hire a video to watch at home. This may have some bearing on the fact that when they hear there is something happening in the town hall tonight, they see a chance for something different just for a change. While this may be apart of the reason why the percentage of the population who attend one of my meetings in a given area can be larger in a smaller community, I feel that it does not account for that different feeling I get as people enter the hall in a place like Bisbee. Of course in a small town, a large proportion already know each other, but in a city they could have come from many different areas and few may ever have met before. This tends to make the meeting a quieter, and one might almost say more sombre gathering, especially during the time people are coming in and taking their seats. They tend to look for a place where there are not a lot of other people already seated. But in the small town they recognise friends sitting there and move in with them, resulting in a babble of voices as they greet each other and discuss what has been going on in their lives amongst themselves.

It may seem strange for me to say that this camaraderie between the members of the public who have gathered together for mutual benefit sets the tone for the evenings proceedings. Something happens within me which tells me this will be a great evening. Words will flow easily from my lips. I know I will be totally at ease with this group of people before me. I seem to know they will be listening keenly to everything I have to say, and taking in whatever I have to tell them.

Meantime, back in the city I am watching a few people straggling in, looking for a place where they can sit where they will not be disturbed by some stranger wanting to speak to them. Sometimes I feel at this stage as if I can almost read the minds of some of them as they look nervously around the hall. I feel they are beginning to have thoughts like, what am I doing here, or I wonder if this is going to be worth the bother of getting here. As the time for me to begin the evenings procedures approaches, I sometimes find myself glancing at the handful of people, usually sitting quietly in their seats, and then walking out the door to take a look up and down the street to see if there are any more cars pulling into the nearest parking lot, or whether they are all cruising on down the road to some other attraction. It can be very difficult to find oneself standing on the stage of a large hall which is all but empty, yet still expected to give out the same message with the same amount of fervour and sincerity as I did a night or two earlier at some packed hall in that little town a few miles away.

But somewhere, deep down within me I have a strange feeling that there is one more very important reason for this situation which we have not yet considered, and it is this which I would like my readers to give some serious thought to. Planet Earth at this time in its evolvement has become a very materialistic place in which to live. They say that money is the root of all evil, and while this may be tending to stretch things a little, I feel it would be advantageous for us to guide our thoughts along that path for a few moments. The city dweller may well be earning, at least in many cases a considerable amount more per week than most of his small town counterparts, and that may sound fine for him. But let us not look at just one side of the coin, for if we turn it over from the side which says income, we will find the other side reads, expenditure.

You may well be saying, so what. But if you look at a few things like the price you are paying for the rent for that flat you are living in, or maybe check out how much a week the interest on that large mortgage you have on that nice house you bought, then you may well find that you are no better off than your country friend after all. On top of all that there are all those extra things it is so easy to squander your hard won funds on in the city whether it be the restaurant down the road where you love to go and indulge yourself, the casino just across town, or the numerous other attractions which can so quickly eat into that weekly income that you soon begin to wonder where it went. I have come to the conclusion that those whose minds are continually filled with these and a thousand other problems of the material world, have little time to give any thought to the higher realms of the Spirit if you wish to put it that way.

I believe that because the mind, or the computer as I usually refer to it, controls every cell in your body, if it is continually filled with the lower frequency thought pattern of materialism, so the vibration of every cell in the body will be lowered, and the body will tend to lack the same vibrant energy of one who has ample time to give more thought to the higher things in life. Is this then the key to what is happening in our two halls. Is that almost depressed feeling which I am often filled with as those few city people come into the hall something which is rubbing off on me as it were, whereas that wonderful feeling of upliftment and contentment which seems to fill our country hall is a product of the higher vibration of those gathered there with their thought pattern vibrating at an increased frequency due to their relative freedom from the continual worry of making ends meet or perhaps just trying to keep up with the Jones's as the city dwellers tend to have to do.

Science has done wonders in many respects, and while in one way I find myself applauding that, there are times when I cannot help but wonder where it will all lead to. When I was a boy, Monday morning was wash day, and it was my job before leaving for school to light the copper fire so that the clothes could be boiled before my hard working mother lifted them out with an old broom handle then laboriously scrubbed each item on a corrugated scrubbing board before carrying them out all dripping wet to hang them on the line, hoping the weather would stay fine long enough for them to dry. Today we throw them in a washing machine, turn a few switches and go back to whatever else we want to do, knowing that when the clothes are clean we will hear a beeping sound which tells us they have been washed and spun, ready for us to spend a few more minutes moving them from washing machine to dryer with no concern as to whether the rain is still falling outside or not.

All of that is fine and I would not like to see it any other way, but it seems that every few months there is some new development which is crying out for us to spend our money on. When my wife and I were married fifty-seven years ago, none of these things existed. We did have a radio, but of course, such things as a TV, a microwave oven, a mower you didn't even have to push in order to cut your lawn, and so many other modern inventions were something you may have found in a book about science fiction. Of course that meant that as long as one of you was a breadwinner then you could manage quite well with so few necessities to be paid for. But today it is a very different story. Even if there are two breadwinners in the family, there are so many different ways of frittering away those extra dollars, that we finish up with more worries than we had way back there. I sometimes wonder to what extent this ever increasing level of materialism will affect the families of tomorrow. Will they have even less time to give thought to the higher things of life as they attempt to find ways of keeping up with the Jones's, and will it become even more difficult for them to get their priorities right.

A busy weekend has just slipped by, and now it is Monday morning as I once again take my place at my desk to pick up my pen and discover what is about to flow from it. As I sat down and began to give some thought concerning where I should begin, it was as if I was suddenly back in the beautiful home I visited yesterday afternoon in a city about sixty miles from my home, and I immediately had the impression that I should record for you here something which took place there. A workshop had been organised for me for 1 p.m, so I arrived there around 12:30 in order to set up my folding healing couch and put out some books and video tapes so that all would be ready when the students arrived. We had about our usual twenty people sitting in a semi-circle in front of me, and I had a very good feeling about this group as I stood up to speak. I usually speak for about an hour at one of these workshops, and then a patient steps up on to the couch and lays down. On this occasion I soon discovered that he had a lot of poison or other unwanted matter in his blood as my hand would hardly move along his leg as I tried to move it from the foot up towards the hip. This meant I was able to invite the first student up to place her hands above the leg and to feel the pressure between her hands building up as she slowly drew them together.

We made a great start, with the first student finding it hard to believe that she could suddenly discover some difficulty in bringing her hands together when there would appear to be no reason why this should be. As is about normal in these classes, there were only two or three who did not consider their hands had met with any great amount of resistance to their movement along the leg, but the majority were quite overwhelmed by their experience. One man in particular, came under a lot of stress as he worked hard to lift a lot of negative energy away from the patient in his cupped hands. I was amazed to see this one working as if he had been doing healing all his life. He was reacting to the negative energy precisely as I would have done myself after all my years of healing thousands of patients. The more so perhaps because while I had met this man on several occasions in the past, I was quite unaware that he had developed the ability to be used as a channel for the healing energy.

What this man did in the closing minutes of yesterday's meeting is the main reason for recording the events here. I had just thanked the people for coming and had asked them to make good use of what they had learned so that many people in the months and years to come would benefit from their new found ability to be healers. Then as the people started to stand up in readiness for returning home, he asked me if I would mind if he said a few words before the meeting closed. I motioned the people to sit back down again, and a little falteringly he began to speak. As near as I can remember, it went something like this. "I would just like you people to know that seventeen years ago I was diagnosed with a serious case of cancer. I was given radiotherapy, but this appeared to be having little effect, I heard about Colin's ability to heal and travelled to Waihi to visit him. I saw him there three times, and on the last occasion he told me I was free of cancer but the doctors gave me one more chemotherapy treatment.

Approximately two years later I had a testicle swell up and ended up in hospital again. After going to theatre for what I thought was only going to be a check to find out what was wrong, I was told when I was returned to the ward that they had removed one testicle. The Oncology Department doctor told me I should have more radiation treatment but I told them I did not want anymore of that.

I have visited Colin a few times since then whenever I felt I needed some more Magnetic Healing. I have changed my lifestyle and consider myself very lucky in that I now have been enlightened to the fact that there is a cure for all ailments other than the pills and medicine a doctor will prescribe for you. About 18 months ago I was directed by my inner thoughts into joining a discussion group who have further enlightened me into new ways of thinking and carrying out Magnetic Healing.

This led me along a path where I now find myself helping other people to free themselves of ailments. I find this extremely interesting to the point where I have given up my job as a truck driver and am doing as much healing as I can. I can only say many thanks to you Colin because I truly believe it was you who freed me of this disease and who has changed my thinking and ways of life and I hope I have become a wiser being".

We appear to have wandered a long way from our travels in Australia, but episodes such as that which took place yesterday are all an important part of a chapter which is designed to show my readers something of the thrilling results which can present themselves when you give your all in pursuit of health and hope for your fellow beings by agreeing to allow your body to be used as a channel for the loveforce. As you enter my healing room there is a small round frame on the wall hanging on a little chain. It was given to me by a grateful patient some years ago, and many of those who have come for healing since then have commented in some way on its simplicity and the beauty of its message. There is a little picture in the frame. It is a painting of a very small girl sitting on a garden seat cuddling tightly in her arms what must be her favourite doll, and the message above her head simply says, "Love is all you need". How true can a statement be? Have you even thought of just what a Heaven on earth we could have here if everyone knew and understood the meaning of the word, but most of all lived by it? I can never quite understand why something so simple appears to be so difficult for so many to grasp, with the result that we still have a planet so dominated by the opposite emotion, with hate bringing about wars which in turn can surely only bring more hate and more suffering for humanity. Surely the time has come for us to lift ourselves above all this, and do our part in helping to spread that simple message of love ever wider.

But back in Brisbane, while we appear to have made a very poor start with so few making the effort to attend our public meeting, we certainly made up for it when word started to run along the old grape vine and people began to realise what my visit to their city was really all about. It was not long before we had several workshops booked up in different areas, and many would be healers went through what some refer to as that amazing experience of feeling for the first time the healing energy flowing from their hands to the patient on the couch. In keeping with the name of this chapter, I will record for you an interesting piece of feedback from those classes which came in some time later from the one who organised my visit to Brisbane.

"Dear Colin, Thank you for a great life–changing experience, not from just me, but also from the many people you touched during your short visit. There are many more "Open parachutes" in Brisbane since you arrived (Minds are like parachutes, they only function when they are open) We are working together and building a network of people who wish to learn more and practise your method. The list is growing and I will keep you informed of our milestones as they are reached. God bless. Love and light."

Surely a card with something like the above written on it says it all. I could tell you in this book that I am travelling to different areas showing many people how easy it is to become a healer, and you could decide for yourself whether I was telling you the truth or just making it all up to make it sound good. But when evidence such as this is produced, and it has come spontaneously without any prompting from me or anyone else, then I am sure you will agree these people do this of their own freewill because they want to put on paper for me to read, something of what they are feeling deep within themselves.

One very short extract from a reader of some of my previous books would appear to be an appropriate way of concluding this record of just a small portion of the feedback which continues to arrive in my letter box.

"I know you have probably heard this thousands of times before, but thanks for writing your books. They have inspired me and humbled me, and helped put everything into place".

It is my humble prayer that this latest effort to record some of my thoughts, beliefs and understandings will continue to, as she and many others have put it, "Inspire" many to make the effort to discover that, perhaps for some, rather elusive, but most important thing of all, TRUTH.

6. SCHOOL OF LIFE

In 1932 I was a twelve year old boy just finishing the last year of my schooling. Eight years from the time I turned five until I left at the end of '32 seemed like a lifetime for one who was never quite the best scholar in the classroom, and like many other children, was there mainly because I knew I had to be whether I liked it or not. Perhaps without really knowing it at the time, there was somewhere deep within me that desire to discover for myself what life is really all about rather than being told what I am expected to do, not unlike a mob of sheep which are herded together and told by two or three barking dogs what is expected of them and which pen they must enter and stand in. Having been corralled into our respective pens or in this case, classrooms, we are then given what would no doubt have been much the same information as last years class had been offered in that same room. In this manner our feet are firmly placed upon the path which we are meant to follow along with those who have gone before.

Please do not get me wrong here. Of course I realise just as well as anyone else that it is very necessary for a child to go to school to learn how to read, to spell, and to write and many other things which he will need to help him to make his way through the life as an adult which lies ahead. And of course when I say him, that automatically translates into him/her, and perhaps someone can come up with one simple word which will cover that anomaly. But what I am really trying to say here, is that looking back over the past 67 years since the day I left that classroom for the last time I have learnt infinitely more concerning what life is really all about than I could have learnt in many more years of schooling.

Personal experience must surely be the greatest teacher of all. Something we actually experience for ourselves, is not second hand knowledge passed onto us. We no longer need to question a statement that has been made to us and wonder whether it is a true one or not, for when we have an experience of our own then we can accept it for what it is, a fact of life.

I remember thinking just yesterday afternoon as I watched my students come up to the patient and place their hands in the area above the problem just how true the above statements really are. I had spent the first hour as I always do telling them what happens when my hand comes up against a negative force which can totally stop its movement along the body. I talked about many instances of this taking place over the years and how, if the problem in the patient was not a serious one but just some little thing which they may not even be aware of, then the amount of resistance to my hand would be very slight. But I also described to them how I would find it impossible to move my hand any further if the patient was suffering from something really serious such as cancer or aids.

The offering of all this information would have been very much like what they had gone through in the years when they sat in school and the teacher told them many things. Just as it was then, so it would have been for them yesterday. Information given, but nothing to prove that the information was truth, or just something the teacher was telling them. Towards the end of that hour I put it to them this way. I told them I was well aware that they need not necessarily believe that everything I had told them was, as we often say, Gospel Truth. I knew I had done nothing to prove to them that the many words I had spoken to them in the last hour were anything more than just that, words. For all they knew they may have been empty words, just spoken to make myself sound like I was someone special. Someone who could place his hands over a body and find the negative areas which would indicate any physical problems in the body.

But of what use would all this have been to them if I had simply told them about this ability of mine to do these things and packed up and gone home. This would have proved nothing to them. It would not have been enough to satisfy them that what I had told them really was the truth. Toward the end of that first hour I told them that what happens on my healing couch is a little bit like the experience one may have with an electric fence, one of those battery or mains powered wires stretched across a farm to give an animal enough of a shock when they touch it to make sure they do not go any further in that particular paddock. I pointed out to them how someone could describe to them what it is like to touch such a fence. They could describe in as much detail as they like the sudden shock one feels through your body as your hand comes into contact with the wire.

All of this would give them some idea of what it must be like to come into contact with such a wire, but it does not mean that they would now know what it feels like. How are they to know whether you are telling them the truth or not? The fact is, of course, they don't. They may well assume that you are, but that is not proof. I told them there is only one way they could ever know for sure whether they had been told the truth or not, and that was from their own experience and not blindly accepting something they had been told. The one and only way of really knowing without any shadow of a doubt whatsoever what it is like to touch an electric fence is to touch it yourself. Then your computer has been programmed for the rest of your life. Many years later when somebody mentions an electric fence you will know exactly what they are talking about. And so it is for the student in my class. I had spent a whole hour describing what I feel when my hand enters that negative energy above the patients body, and related to them some of the more spectacular results of making contact with that energy. But now the time had come for them to discover for themselves that which I had assured them really was the truth. They had spent their time in school, in this case a whole hour of it, listening to the teacher. But had they really learnt anything, or were they just sitting there wondering whether what they had heard could be proved to be the whole truth and nothing but the truth.

The lady sitting at one end of the half circle of people in front of me looked startled as I turned toward her and suggested we would start with her and make our way to the other end one at a time. She had that sort of look on her face which seemed to be saying, "Why me". I jokingly said, "That will teach you to be on the end of the line won't it" As she sidled up beside me nervously, I told her that at this moment there was only three people in the room. Just you and me and the patient. I suggested she should forget there was anyone else there and together we were going to help the man in front of us laying on the couch hoping for a miracle. After showing her where to put her hands, I removed mine and watched her replace them with her own. I then told her to very slowly begin to bring them together to a central point between them. This is always the interesting part for me, watching for the reaction of the student as her hands begin to enter the problem area. On a few occasions there is little or none, and a disappointed student returns to her seat. But fortunately that is very much the rarity rather than the rule. And this particular occasion was certainly not one of those. That soon became very obvious as her hands began to shake a little and as always, turned red.

You may remember that in chapter three I mentioned how I had asked Dr

Anderson in Vermont about the changing colour of the hands as they enter the negative energy and he told me that it was to do with the corpuscles filling with blood. And here again was that positive proof that already something was happening to the body standing beside me. Yet here was one who assured me she knew nothing about healing and had never before even considered for one moment that she would be able to feel anything in the energy field of another body. But it was very soon obvious that she was coming under quite a lot of stress as she gathered together a heavy load of the unwanted dross from the patient and slowly but deliberately lifted it away in her cupped hands.

With this one being the first student to come up and try her hand at being used as a channel for the universal energy, I felt we had made an excellent start, and that this would tend to give the rest of the group more confidence. I reckoned they would be thinking that if she could do it so well on her very first try, then maybe it would work for them too. And work it did, as one after another they stood beside the couch to take their turn at proving that what I had spent an hour telling them was indeed the truth. I had spent that hour talking to them as any teacher may do, but this was different. This was a practical hands on experience. I did not need to tell them anything more. They were programming their own computers now in their own way, and not relying on someone trying to explain something to them in mere words.

At last they had reached out and touched the electric fence for themselves and no one needed to tell them what it was like anymore. Now they really knew. And they knew that anytime, any place where they may be confronted with someone who was ill and needed healing, they would be able to place their hands in that ones energy field or aura as it is perhaps more commonly referred to, and feel the area where the problem in the physical body was reflected in that aura. It is difficult for me to put on paper just how I feel at a time like this. It is a wonderfully satisfying experience to watch each one discover their true potential and to see the joy which so obviously fills them as they realise the importance of what is taking place in their lives.

Here they are back in school again. Learning something new. But not just being told that this is so, or this is what you should believe because I believe it. Oh no, this is a very different school. It is the school of life. The school of personal experience. This is a school where there can be no doubts. Where no one need wonder any longer whether they are being faced with truth or just being lectured about some phenomena which they have no positive proof about. But as I watch the face of each one as their hand begins to feel the pressure in front of it, I know that in many cases their minds are in turmoil. I know they are thinking something like, "Oh my God, it really does work for me. I can't believe this. I can hardly bring my hands together. "I know this is the sort of thought pattern which is racing around in their confused minds, because while some of them bite their lip and just push doggedly on with the job of lifting the dross away, some of them speak those thoughts out loud for all to hear.

And how do I know how they feel about what is happening at this time? Well as I have just mentioned, some of them make no secret of it by speaking their thoughts. But this is not the only proof I have of how this experience affects them. There are many who, while they may say little or nothing while it is actually happening, sit down at some later date and express their gratitude to me for having allowed them to learn another valuable lesson in the school of life. Some do it by phone while others use the pen. So perhaps I should record for you one or two short extracts from some of these letters or cards which they send to me in order to pass on to me their feelings concerning what they have learnt.

"Dear Colin, A note to say thank you for the talk and workshops you took in our town last weekend. Feedback has been very positive and everyone is keen to meet again this weekend, which I have already organised. Only good things can come from your teaching and I know our town will be a better place for it?"

And from another area, "I am writing to thank you for a wonderful afternoon at Lorraine's place and sharing a meal with you. Since that day our group has practised healing with great results. We are grateful for all you taught us."

While I am watching the reaction each one shows as they approach that area in the aura, I am not just wondering what may be going on in that ones mind, I am looking far away into the future and visualising what is taking place in front of me. I am thinking of all the people who will gain at some time from what I see happening. It may be next week, it may be next year, but if this one who has discovered her latent ability to heal continues to use this throughout the rest of her life as I know many are doing, then it may be that years from now when the time allotted for me to remain in this body has come to an end, I will look down from the real world, the world of higher vibration, or Spirit if you wish, and revel in the joy it will bring me as I watch her putting out her hands again to bring relief to an ailing brother or sister of Planet Earth.

And just a little more proof that this will be so. An extract from a letter from the South Island of NZ where I visited to open their minds a few years ago runs like this. "We absolutely enjoy the healing, and are very grateful for the gift. We have some very good successes, perhaps our best being cervical cancer cured. Two tests in the hospital confirmed it. We are thanking you again for teaching us. You made such a big difference to our life". I think I have already mentioned that the word "Inspire" or its derivatives keep coming up in my correspondence, and here again is another example.

"I am so glad my friend asked you to come to see us in our city here. Even though the subjects you covered in your talks are very familiar and accepted in my family, you have inspired me to spread the message and I am more motivated than ever before to do good work and "Zap" with universal healing energy all those who would consent. I have never felt entirely comfortable asking for money for the massage or reflexology I have been doing. But I really like the idea of the choice for people to make a donation if they are able. Your workshop would not have been accessible to me if it had required more money than I was able to pay, I now feel like I have walked into the tunnel of light, and my world or my reality has changed. Oh, the possibilities. I am so excited. Thank you Colin". Yes, the possibilities indeed. They are endless.

Cervical cancers on one hand, to a child having six or seven epileptic fits a day on the other. These and many more are the rewards one receives for opening the mind to those endless possibilities which are available when we have the courage to step outside the inhibiting boundaries of a negative low frequency vibration science which refuses to look right or left in case it should be faced with something which does not fit into its narrow path of preconceived ideas.

These last words were written at 11 pm last night before switching off the light and getting myself some sleep. Perhaps it is just another one of those strange coincidences yet again, but before picking up my pen this morning I spent a little time looking through the news paper which had just arrived in the box. I turned over the first page, and there on the next was a headline above a short news item. It read, "School too stifling." Being in the middle of a chapter titled "The school of life " I decided to read it to see what their research had come up with. While I feel it did not tell me much which I did not already know, it did seem that it had been designed to fit in very snugly with some of the statements I made a little earlier in this chapter.

"Five year olds cannot wait to start school, but quickly find it a letdown, and a "sausage factory" school system could be to blame." Eileen Ledger, a researcher at the University of Otago's Centre for children, said that in many ways the school system stifled free thinking and was full of rules designed to suit teachers, not children". Stifled free thinking? Perhaps not quite the same words I used to describe my time at school in the opening paragraphs of this chapter, but certainly near enough to the same general thought pattern concerning what she referred to rather more bluntly than I was prepared to do, as the "Sausage factory school system".

I have long since come to realise that unless we make the effort to go out and search for truth, then it is most unlikely we will ever discover very much of it. But another letter in the mail a few weeks ago shows once again how more and more people are making that effort, and more importantly, recognising truth when they see it. It is one thing to be faced with the truth, but it is a very different thing to be able to say to yourself, this is it, and really know within yourself that it is so. For me, something happens inside of me when I come up against a statement which has that unmistakable ring of truth about it. While it is difficult to put this into words, perhaps the nearest I could come to it would be to say that there is a tingling feeling which flows through me, and I know this is it.

"Dear Mr Lambert, I was delighted when my thirteen year old daughter brought home a pile of books from the library to find your first book "WHY" amongst them. I read it eagerly, then set about finding your next book "HERES WHY", only to find there is just one copy left in our city library - kept in safe keeping – not for issue. However, I am now reading "YOU TOO CAN HEAL" with great interest. My only regret is that I did not discover these books earlier. Thank you so much for taking the time during your very busy life to share your learnings and wisdom through your books. Thank you also for writing in a way that can be so easily understood. For me they have restored a feeling of hope in a world where hope has become a word from the past".

Can you even begin to imagine how humbling for me letters such as this can be. As I read them on their arrival at my home, I am filled once again with that exhilarating inner feeling of gratitude in the knowledge that the untold hours of searching for truth, then having recognised it, passed it onto others through the medium of the pen has once again produced dividends way beyond anything I could have dreamed of at the time my search began. The fruits of ones labour can be judged by the effect which is created on ones fellow beings, and mail like this tells me in no uncertain terms that my efforts to bring onto Planet Earth, in this its hour of need, a little more of the light of understanding, have not gone unnoticed.

I sometimes sit and think about people who spend their lives and make a living from doing things like writing horror stories, making films or videos filled with violence or pornography. Or those who place on the Internet the recipe for making a bomb, knowing full well that they can guarantee the end result will be some young person following those instructions with disastrous results. Others spend their lives inventing bigger, and dare I say, better ways, of creating mass destruction, be it a land mine, a bombing plane or an atom bomb. I think they call these people "Inventors". Surely a misnomer if ever there was one.

Can one such as this really gain any satisfaction from his incarnation, knowing that his efforts throughout his life have brought nothing but unbelievable suffering and death to many of his brothers and sisters. I find it hard to imagine just how these ones manage to sleep, particularly after they see the results of their labours displayed on their TV screen. Do they watch the screaming women and children running for their lives in an attempt to escape, all too often the inescapable, then proudly say to themselves, I was responsible for that. I was the one who invented that new weapon. Will the wonders of a negative destructive science ever cease?

I am sorry but somehow my mind refuses to comprehend how this can be. How can any human being enjoy all the things he is able to buy with the big money he is paid for producing these death dealing weapons of total destruction, designed to do nothing else but massacre indiscriminately his fellow beings? I presume these people receive letters also concerning the work they have done. I assume they would receive a letter of commendation from perhaps the munitions factory or even the Government thanking them for doing such a good job of inventing this latest weapon, but for me, I would much rather receive one like the one this short extract came from, one which was sent by a man and his wife who I had shown the art of Magnetic Healing to two or three years ago.

"The healing guides are working more through us now, and my husband is channelling the energy in the identical way to you. We are also happy to teach people how to heal. We had three at our home today and they are now keen to practise. The healing opens up a new world for us and we find it very rewarding to work in this way". I know which letter I would rather have the pleasure of receiving, and it is certainly not the first one of those two. Surely carrying with you through life a lighted torch and using it to light even a candle here and a candle there must be infinitely more rewarding than carrying a snuffer in order to use it to snuff out each light you find burning, and by so doing, bring the world into darkness.

At this point I would like to ask you, my reader, which one you are carrying and whether you feel totally satisfied with your burden. Do you lay your head on the pillow each night with a clear conscience quite satisfied that you have made the best possible use of the hours you have been given, or did you simply fritter them away doing nothing really useful? Nothing which would have helped to make Planet Earth even a tiny weeny bit better place for those who will follow in your footsteps in the years to come. Or did you use your time to do something even worse. Did you even in some small way make life more difficult for someone, or maybe even many. Did your aura shine today with the light of your love for your fellowman, or did dark thoughts of hate, malice or vengeance toward him cast a shadow that blotted out your light?

You and you alone are the one who really knows the answers to these questions, but perhaps even more importantly, you are the only one who can do anything about brightening your light if it has become dimmed. Do remember that everything begins for you in that wonderful computer we have been given. What you will do with your time and with your energy will depend entirely on how you have programmed it. You are what you believe, and your actions will be no more than a reflection of that belief. If you think the world owes you a living as they say, and you are going to get it no matter who gets hurt on the way, then your light is going to be very dim indeed. There are far more than enough of those ignorant individuals polluting our planet with their low frequency destructive thought pattern, and if you are one of them then it is time to change. Time to recognise your true soulself within. Time to raise your conscious awareness of your duty toward your fellowman and the part you should be playing to bring into being the wonderful new age of light and enlightenment. As far away as it may seem, it is not a hopeless dream. It can be achieved, but only when you do your part in bringing it about.

The number of people who are coming to a new realisation of the necessity of learning lessons from the school of life, then putting those lessons to good use in pursuit of health, hope and upliftment of body mind and soul is slowly rising as more and more people realise that we cannot continue to abuse Mother Earth and her children in the way we have been doing since "Science" first made it possible for us to do so. There has always been wars throughout history when man wielded sword or bow and arrow against his fellowman in his ignorance, not knowing that to hurt another is to hurt yourself because you are all one. But at least these skirmishes were no more than a pinprick would be on an elephant's hide compared to the mass destruction of a Hiroshima or a Nagasaki. But even these were minute compared to what the "Advancement" of science has so proudly prepared for us today. 'Bigger and Better' seems to be the catchcry.

In our stupidity we say we must have more and better weapons because that other country has some new ones. That one has nuclear capability so we must have it too. Surely the simple answer would be for each country to destroy all of their weapons, as the Bible puts it, turn their swords into plough shears, then no one need to be a threat to anyone. Perhaps that is just too simple an answer to a problem that need not exist apart from the fact that the manufacture of munitions in their many forms on a worldwide scale has to be one of the largest moneymaking occupations on the planet. Fear, one of mankind's greatest enemies still stalks the planet, but it can only do so for as for as long as we allow it to. Change hate and mistrust for love and understanding and fear will dissolve away like a snowman in the sun.

Life is for living, but it is also for learning. We all make mistakes in our life. No one is perfect yet, but must we be so blind as to continue to make the same mistakes over and over as we have been doing for so long. We must learn by our mistakes as we make our way through the school of life, and make sure we do not repeat them. From my experience in the field of healing during the past thirty years, the medical profession in the main seems to be content to continue to do exactly that. Change can never come while other possibilities are ignored. The doctor who assures me she would never believe that I could possibly do anything for anybody by waving my hands over a body, has of course never seen me work and is not aware that I am actually passing my hands through an energy surrounding the body and diagnosing the areas where that field has become out of phase.

She probably does not even know there is a field around a body. She was taught for several years about the physical body and learned a lot about the organs and their various functions, but as one open minded doctor told me, he was never taught anything about an energy field. My lady doctor probably imagines I say abracadabra or chant something as my hands are, as she puts it, being waved over the body. The reason she has not seen how I work of course is not because I refused to show her. Far from it. I would have liked nothing better than to have been able to demonstrate Magnetic Healing to her, or better still shown her how she could do the same if she wished. But of course as I am sure we all know, there are none so blind as those who do not wish to see. And yes, she was one of those. The closed mind, believing that she already knew that her way, the way she had spent so much time and energy and money learning about was the only way.

But as you have seen in an earlier chapter we do have the Dr Andersons of Vermont and others of similar openness who are prepared to look and to listen and learn from that most valuable school of all, the school of life. Consider for instance the content of one more letter which I will now quote to you from. "Dear Mr Lambert, Our family with four children came to NZ a few years ago. We emigrated from Germany and lived for more than one year in the South Island. The first book we discovered in a bookshop there was your book, "You Too Can Heal". We both studied it carefully and were deeply impressed by the message". You may be saying, "So what, it is obvious you receive many letters along these lines as you have already quoted from some of them." That is very true but there was something very different about this one as you will now see as I copy the next few lines.

"My husband is a medical doctor (Paediatrician and Surgeon) and he is originally from Armenia. I decided to write to you these lines because it could be satisfactory for you to know that there are existing people like him who would value and accept your thoughts. We would like to ask you to send your previous book "Magnetic Healing and Other Realities' for which I have enclosed a cheque."

I am not quite sure now how many beats my heart missed when I read that passage, but I know it was a wonderful moment for me when I realised here was a man who had trained for many years as a paediatrician and a surgeon who was prepared to admit that he, as his wife had put it, valued and accepted my thoughts. Yes, the times they are achanging, and that change can only be for the better as more people find the courage to learn their lessons well and to make good use of their newfound knowledge.

We can lift ourselves above the ignorance of the past which has kept us chained to the dogmatic teaching of a hide bound science, ever afraid to step outside the boundaries they have set for others to follow. I am aware that I have probably mentioned in one of my other books an article which was printed in the Financial Review in 1986, but for those of you who have not had the opportunity to read it, I would like to repeat it here to prove to you that when I speak of scientists having boundaries which they refuse to pass through, I am not doing so without some substantial evidence with which to back up my statement.

"Scientists do not condemn the theories of doctor Bevan Reid, but they do comment however, that his ideas are well outside the traditional boundaries of science. Dr Reid, a lecturer in obstetrics and gynaecology at the University of Sydney admits the reaction to his theories is often "Total disbelief", and that they are ignored by his peers. But he believes he has the evidence from repeated experiments to prove there is an electromagnetic force surrounding all living matter, and that this force can induce changes in cells without chemical interaction".

The first time I read this statement I could hardly believe what I was reading for several reasons. For a start I could not imagine why it had been printed in, of all publications, the Financial Review. A Medical journal perhaps, or a New Age publication, or even some ordinary magazine which does print all sorts of general knowledge, but not the prestigious Financial Review. But there it was anyway, and a very interesting contribution to any publication. An electromagnetic force surrounding all living matter. Sometimes I think the wonders of science will never cease. How did he ever manage to make such a wonderful discovery? And what is this electromagnetic force he is enthusing about? Surely he cannot be talking about the energy which I have been photographing with that Kirlian machine I mentioned having had made for me in chapter four. The same energy which I have been working through to bring new health to thousands of patients, both man and beast, for the past thirty years. Yes, obviously one and the same.

Why then, as a respected scientist who has come up with something different after repeated experiments would his colleagues ignore him? Would it not be more logical to spend some time following up those experiments to find out for themselves whether those statements are true or false? How could science expect to advance if, instead of doing that, they simply cast off his claims as being "Outside the traditional boundaries of science" . My simple question to any scientist would be to ask him why he must insist on having any boundaries in what he is prepared to investigate. Surely the old "Unless you can see it, weigh it, or put it in a bottle" sort of attitude should have been dispensed with long ago.

I have had to learn the hard way over the years that the reason why I have not been able to get through to most medical people the fact that Magnetic Healing really does work, is because to use it one has to step well outside those traditional boundaries of orthodox science. How can they explain how cells in a body which have become "out of phase" making the body what we call ill, can be put back into phase again so that the body is then at ease, instead of diseased without the practitioner even touching his patient? Of course the simple answer to that question is, they can't, and they never will, as long as they insist on remaining within their strict boundaries. But as Nicola Tesla once said, "In that single decade when science first begins to investigate the non physical, they will make more progress in that decade than science has made in the past century".

Of course for the average medic it is bad enough when Dr Reid says there is an electromagnetic force surrounding all living matter, but to suggest that this energy can actually be used to "Induce changes in cells without chemical interaction" must surely be little short of heresy. However, I sometimes wonder who is the most upset by this statement. Is it the doctor or the multimillion dollar drug companies. Perhaps this is the real reason why we have heard no more discussion on this subject since the story was first published in 1986. To use the universal energy which is everywhere and is free to any who wish to use it certainly means that everytime someone does use it to heal an ailing body, that one no longer needs to continue to visit his doctor every now and then with his cheque book in his hand. But I have a feeling that it is even more important that if he is not visiting his doctor, then the doctor is not writing out a prescription for one or other of the drugs those companies make.

Yes, without chemical interaction. No chemicals, no drugs of any kind being put into the patients body means no profit, but listen well when I tell you that it also means no nasty side effects. And what a blessing that can be for the patient. I have lost count of the number of patients I have seen laying on my couch with a very bald looking head after having been given chemotherapy for cancer. At such times I can not help thinking this is the visible damage to the body, but how much invisible damage must there be hidden away inside the body. This one did not have cancer in his hair, so why would you want to do something which would remove a perfectly good head of hair. It is extremely unlikely this will be the only damage to the cells of that body, and yet if this one had been treated in the first place with the totally non-toxic loveforce energy, the only cells which would have been affected in any way would have been the ones which had become out of phase and needed to be restored to normality or removed from the body to make room for new ones.

In these cases as I work hard to restore the body to its normal state, I can not help wondering how much of my time and energy and effort is going into removing or restoring those cells which have been affected by the imbalance to which we have given the name, cancer, and how much of it is being used to undo the damage which is the direct result of the chemicals given to the body. In a little book by the name of "Radionics" written by David Tansley we find this statement. "We are rapidly entering the era of the mind (what I often refer to as the computer) and even now as we look at some of its remarkable capacities, it is evident that the human mind is a thing of awesome power with abilities and capacities we have barely begun to tap. These of course, when harnessed and guided by the highest motives, can be used to heal and bring harmony to life in many unusual ways, often in cases where all else has failed."

Abrams, the father of Radionics, discovered the principles of electronic medicine. He established through his researches that diseases were vibratory energy states, and could be treated with energy, whether in the form of homoeopathic or by electromagnetic means. I do not know whether David Tansley has ever seen the article from the Financial Review, but I am sure he would applaud Dr Reids statement concerning the discovery of an electromagnetic force surrounding all living matter, and the use of this energy to induce changes in cells without chemical interaction. As I come across an ever increasing number of similar statements being made by different people from scattered areas around the planet, I begin to feel within me that the single decade when science will first begin to investigate the non-physical is almost upon us.

7. ABSENT HEALING

When I am speaking to a group of people whether it be in a hall at a public meeting, or a smaller workshop in someone's home, I very often make this statement. I have found that if I try to tell some medical people that when I have an ailing body on a couch in front of me I can run my hand through the energy field surrounding it and find out exactly where the source of their problem is without them telling me anything, they look at me very strangely. I get the feeling they are thinking I must be mad to believe that anyone could do that. But of course if I should happen to be stupid enough to say to them, actually I do not need to have the physical body there, it does not matter if they are in New York or London, as long as I have their name and their request for healing, I will pick up the problems on that body just the same.

Then their look turns to one of pity for some deluded individual who is crazy enough to believe that he can do what everyone knows is the impossible. It would be difficult for me to convince them that the 'impossible' happens quite frequently for me, and what is more, I have plenty of proof to prove it. We have been talking a lot about the electromagnetic energy which surrounds every living thing, and the interaction between those energies. When a healer places his hand over a body and turns his computer to the desired frequency of transmission of energy, then that energy interacts with the energy surrounding his patient. Just how it will react will depend on a number of things, and in this chapter it is my desire to attempt to bring to my readers some of the conclusions I have come to during 30 years of time and something like 35 to 40 thousand patients.

While there are still many things which I do not fully understand by any means concerning this amazing phenomenon, I do feel that it is my duty to pass on anything I have learned during those years, to any one who has an open enough mind to accept it. I am well aware there are still many who would not consider the information I will pen here to be worth a second look. But then, I realise that any such as those will not even bother to take a first look anyway, leave alone a second. But that will be their loss, and a gain I hope for those who do.

Several years ago while travelling through another part of the country I called in to the home of a man I had met two or three times before. He was a very good healer, but was also well known as a diviner of water and oil. We sat down with a cup of coffee and talked about many things, but mostly our interest in healing. He was one of those, who like myself, receive requests for healing from many areas, and during discussion of his ability to work in this way, he suddenly stood up and walked over to a cupboard and opened the door. In doing so he exposed to my view a large stack of letters, piled one upon another on the shelves.

I remember thinking that there appeared to be something strange about this because they did not appear to have been opened. I thought he was going to bring one or two of them out for me to see, but he stopped short of that, and merely pointed towards them from a foot or so away. At this stage he turned to face me and said "You see all those letters there, they are from people who have written to me for absent healing, but I dare not pick one of them up, because if I did, the moment I touched it I would automatically start giving out healing to the writer of that particular letter. This would put my body under a certain amount of stress, and as you know, I am now in my eighties and feel that my time for doing that work has come to and end".

Absent healing? Yes that was a whole new level of absent healing for me. I have to open the letter, find the persons name, then ask for that one to be placed on the couch in front of me to allow me to visualise the body there and work on it just as I would if it was there in the physical form. But here was a man who had developed his sensitivity to the low frequency vibration of a group of cells which had become out of phase that he automatically began to work to put those cells back into phase again without him even being aware of the name of the one who had written to him requesting him to return the cells of their body to their normal state.

If I have such extreme difficulty in convincing followers of orthodox science that I can help someone who is ill by placing the etheric form of that one on my couch, then what possible chance would one have of getting through to them the fact that here was one who could do that without even knowing the name of his patient or whether she was at the time of healing, living in New Zealand or some faraway country. I have always considered that the only way it would be possible to give someone absent healing, would be by looking at the name of your patient as it has been written on a piece of paper, and by so doing your wonderful computer is automatically tuned to the particular frequency of the owner of that name.

People often ask me what would happen if there were two people with precisely the same name living in the same area, and would I possibly work on the wrong one by mistake. There is one rule concerning absent healing which I have tried to stick with fairly rigidly. If someone asks me to work on their friend Mary Jones who is not very well, my response to that request is to ask them whether Mary Jones has requested me to do so. I do not feel I have the right to work on someone who has not asked me to help them. There are many people who would not come near my healing room, either because they know it would be a waste of time, or due to their particular religious beliefs they would not allow me to use Satan to try to heal them.

I feel that when someone requests me to give them healing either by writing to me, or speaking to me on the telephone, then that one has put out on to the ethers a vibration which does not just stay with them, but becomes part of the "all that is" which surrounds the planet. If there should happen to be two Mary Jones's in the same area, then one of them will have put out this thought pattern to the ethers, and the other will not have done so. Hence there will only be one request for healing out there, so that is the one my computer will be tuning in to.

But in my friends case, this ability had obviously been fine tuned to the stage where by touching the letter which contained the patients requests for healing, he was automatically tuning in to the thought pattern she had created as she wrote the letter. You could say that in this respect he was practising what is commonly referred to as Psychometry, Oxford dictionary describes this ability as "the supposed divination of facts about events, people etc from inanimate objects associated with them". I am happy to give Oxford the prize for that explanation. Like probably everyone else on this kindergarten planet we call Earth, they are not able to explain how anyone achieves Psychometry, but do give a good idea of what it is even if they cover themselves against the possibility of being told they are naive to consider this could take place, by using the words "supposed divination".

It would appear to be quite clear to me that this is precisely what my friend was doing. By touching a letter which had been written by someone needing assistance for a health problem, his computer was automatically psychometrising that "inanimate object" which was associated with one who wrote it. Many times I have seen other people, often at a meeting of mediums where one of them has been handed an object such as a ring or watch without being told who the object belongs to. The owner will have removed a ring for instance, put in an envelope and placed it on a tray herself so that no one else's vibration would interfere with hers. This is always done before the Psychometrist enters the room, so that she can have no idea who the object belongs to. She will then pick it up and by tuning into the vibration of its owner with which the object is filled, and surrounded, she will begin to describe what she sees or feels.

It can be very interesting to see the reaction of the owner when the Psychometrist comes up with some pertinent details concerning his or her life which there could be no way she could have been aware of. I am aware that the sceptics will say it had all been pre-arranged, but there have been too many times when I have known for certain that the owner of the ring and the one doing the psychometry had never met, and there was no way she could have known any of the details she came up with.

While watching an Australian documentary one evening, I saw something which made me give some thought to the possibility that, like the ability to be a healer which I am finding almost everyone appears to have laying dormant within them, waiting to be recognised, this faculty we refer to as psychometry may also be a part of our natural ability which we in the so-called civilised world have lost. There is an old saying "use it or lose it" and it would seem to be this is what has taken place in this case.

What the documentary showed was some police attempting to find someone who had been lost in Outback Australia. The terrain was extremely rough and rocky, and try as they might, they could find no clue whatsoever which may help them to discover the direction in which the lost one may have travelled. They finally decided it was quite hopeless, as there was no way he would have left any footmarks on such rocky ground. Then someone had a bright idea. They decided to ask a black aborigine tracker to see if he would be able to give any assistance to the white police who were becoming desperate as they realised the unfortunate lost one could not last long in the extremely hot and dry conditions.

A tracker was soon found and brought to the area where the police had lost the trail. It was quite an education to watch this elderly black man who looked as if he was not far removed from the Stone Age, and to see how quickly he picked up the direction in which he said the missing person had travelled. Every now and then he would stop and look at a stone which looked like any other stone. But somehow he knew that this stone had been stood on by the wanderer. They moved across that bleak looking country stone by stone for quite some distance until they finally found their man in a bad state, but good enough to be able to be taken back to civilisation and restored to normal health.

At the time of watching this documentary I was at a total loss to understand how anyone's eyesight could be so much better than all of the police and helpers on the job, that he was able to see marks on bare stones that no one else was aware of. But looking back at that now I have a feeling that he was not seeing any marks on certain stones at all, but was psychometrising the ones which the man they were looking for had placed one of his feet on as he passed that way. Could he have left on those stones his particular vibration which was being picked up by the tracker, in the same way that psychometrist was tuning in to the specific vibration of the owner of the ring. Your guess is as good as mine, but it would certainly not surprise me at all if this turns out to be the answer to the uncanny capability of these people. Is this something which all people have laying dormant and untouched, waiting for us to recognise these inherent gifts which we have refused to use for so long that we have ceased to realise they even exist.

I would like to take you back now to our elderly healer in his lounge with this cupboard full of unopened letters. Just as I was about to leave his home that day, he asked me to step into another room where he wished to conduct a short experiment. As I came in I saw him pick up a pair of what are commonly called L wires. They are well named because that is precisely what they are. Two pieces of fairly stiff wire, which have been bent into the shape of the letter L. When used for divining of any kind the short end is held in the hand while the long end points forward away from the operator and they are kept parallel to each other, a few inches apart. The diviner can use them in this way while searching for such things as water, oil or minerals of some kind. He can also use them mentally to ask all sorts of questions. If the answer to the question you are asking your innerself is yes, then the wires will cross, but if it is no then they will part. At least that is the way they work for me and I think for most people I have seen using them.

But today I was to see something very different as this incredibly sensitive elderly man demonstrated his skill to me. He asked me to stand in front of him about three feet away, then he took the L wires in his hands and pointed them toward me. He then said he wanted to measure the extent of my aura to see how far it extended from my body. He explained that he had tried this a number of times with different people and had discovered that they could vary quite a lot, with some auras only extending a short distance from the body and others several feet or more. When the wires had settled down with no movement as they pointed at my body he told me he would start counting from one foot and go on to two feet etc, and when he reached the distance to which my aura extended, the wires would part and this would tell him the extent of my aura.

The counting began and he had soon reached ten, eleven, twelve feet. He looked a little puzzled as he continued to count to an even higher number and the wires refused to move. I felt he was becoming a little concerned and was wondering whether perhaps just as he would not pick up one of those envelopes any more because his body was not capable of being used in that way for healing any longer, perhaps he should not be doing this experiment. I began to think that maybe he had finally lost all of his ability to do any form of divining whether it was checking for a problem on a body or calculating the extent of someone's aura. And then it happened. Having become tired of counting the distance from my body to the end of my aura, foot by foot, he took the bull by the horns as they say and said in a loud clear voice "infinity?" I thought he looked a little shocked as the wires flew apart and almost wrapped themselves around him.

As he gained his composure he began to tell me how he had tried doing this on quite a lot of people and this was only the second time he had need to resort to saying 'infinity' before he could get any response. He then said "I suppose you are aware this means your aura does not stop. It makes a complete circuit of the planet, and so you would be able to work on anyone on the other side of the planet just as easily as if the person was here with you".

How much there is for us to learn. I often say that the more I learn the more I realise I know almost nothing. Creation does not give up its secrets lightly; they have to be earned. They are not handed to you on a plate willy nilly. Too many people would not just use them, but would abuse them, and bring unwanted destruction to Mother Earth and her children. I believe that it is only as you make the effort to raise your conscious awareness of your true soulself within and recognise your oneness with all that is that your vibratory rate is raised to that elevated level where you become one with the higher understanding and mystery begins to be revealed as knowledge.

Although I still know very little about the modus operandi of absent healing, I do know that it works, and that it can work very well. There have been at least two occasions I can recall when I have been at a meeting where there have been what we commonly refer to as a medium channelling their guide. On one of these I asked the guide how it was that I had discovered that I did not need to have the physical body in front of me, but could just visualise that ones body being there and work on it just the same providing the patient had asked me to do so. This was very soon after I had first realised this was possible, and so had only tried it a few times, but already felt that it was working well judging by the enthusiastic reports received from the patients.

The guide listened to my question, then slowly said "Well, you know, when I look at your work I think you probably do an even better job when you do not have the physical body getting in your way". This was not quite what I had expected as an answer. I had asked the question in the hope of having described to me that modus operandi I have just stated I know so little of. While I cannot remember the rest of his answer in his words, I do know that it was along the lines of not worrying about how it works, but just knowing that it does. And this is where the parting of the ways really begins between any of us who use our hands to heal the sick whether we be doing it directly on the physical body or absently.

Science as we know it must feel that they understand every detail of the whys and wherefores of everything they do. They appear to be stuck with some strange dogmatic law that says, "If you don't understand the method by which this is supposed to take place, then it will not work". I have long since realised that statement is far from being a true one. Many times in my workshops I have told my students not to be concerned about the healing they are about to learn how to do, actually works, but just to believe that it does, and it will. I seem to hear that great Master teacher they call Jesus saying, "Except ye believe". He did not say to his disciples that they would not be able to do healing as he did unless they understood exactly how it happened, but he did tell them to believe. Then it would become a matter of "These things shall ye do, and greater things than these".

And with his permission I would like to repeat those words to any of my readers who may have a desire to become a healer. Just believe; just know that if you ask to be used as a humble channel for his love force then it will be granted. If your desire in this way is sincere, then yes, these things shall ye do.

I must admit I was a little surprised to hear the guide suggesting that he thought I would probably do a better job by not having the body in the way.

I had never thought of it that way, and even now, if the patient does not live too far away, I still like to have him on the couch in front of me if possible. Perhaps it is partly because I like to be able to talk to my patients as I work on them, and hopefully be able to give someone who may have a serious problem such as cancer, a little extra hope by telling them about some of the cancer patients I have worked on very successfully in the past, so that they will know the negative message, like only having a few weeks to live, which doctors all too often convey to their patients, is not necessarily true after all.

But of course if the patient lives on the other side of the world or even in Australia, then I am happy to work on that one absently, and know that the work will be done just as well if not "even better" as the guide had suggested. I certainly do find that it never takes as long to clear the negative energy from a patient if I am doing it in this way, so perhaps this is part of what he meant by doing a better job without having the physical body in the way.

The other occasion I can recall at this time took place under very similar circumstances. I was part of a group of people in a meeting where we were discussing our healing work, when one of the group informed me that her friend who was too ill to come to the meeting had requested her to ask me if I would give her some absent healing. This form of healing was quite new to me at the time, and all of those which I had worked on in this way had been done in my healing room where I had stood beside my couch and asked for the etheric counterpart of the sick one's body to be placed there for me to work on.

My response in this case was to say to the one who had made the request for healing for her friend "But I don't have a couch to put her on, there is not even a table here or we could use that". Sitting to one side was a medium whose guide was apparently watching the proceedings and listening to our conversation. As I finished that sentence, I was really taken aback by a loud clear voice coming through the medium from her guide. He said "Why do you need a couch or a table she doesn't weigh anything".

Wow! That was an angle I hadn't even considered, but when you think about it, he was so right, she doesn't weight anything, she is energy, in one of its many forms of frequency of vibration. She is not the body, she is the lifeforce which animates the body and gives the physical form life. We could take a length of wire and weigh it and yes it would have weight, in the same way that if you were to weigh a corpse it too would have weight, but be a lifeless object, because the lifeforce had left it. If you had weighed it a little earlier before that lifeforce left it at the point of time we so vaguely refer to as death, then it would still have registered on the scale just the same. If we were to connect our length of wire which we have just weighed, to a 230-volt electrical system, it would still weigh the same even though now we would find it to be a very lively object if we were to touch it.

So here we have from our guide a very interesting fact. Since realising this I have found that if there is no table or couch available to place the lifeforce on, then yes, I can just stand anywhere in a room, put out my hands in front of me and ask for Mary Smith to be placed there and visualise her floating there. My hand will come up against resistance when it reaches the area where the problem is exactly the same as it would if her etheric lifeforce was on a table or if the physical counterpart was there. I know it begins to sound a little bit like science fiction, but I can assure you that everything I have said here has been proven to me many times by the letters and the phone calls received from grateful patients. The case I mentioned in Chapter 4 where I received a letter from a man in Vancouver who was very ill with cancer, and within two months was sending me airline tickets for a return flight to his home because of the relief from pain which he had received when I gave him healing from my home in New Zealand was a typical example. But there have been many more, and perhaps the story of a man who was in a wheelchair due to having cancer in the lower part of his spine would be an interesting one to relate.

Originally he was wheeled into my healing room and we had some difficulty in lifting him onto the couch as he was a fairly large man and my couch is quite high to enable me to keep my back as straight as possible while working. He felt that he had quite a lot of relief from his first healing and was keen to return for more even though he had to travel almost 100 miles each way. Many people have very different reactions to the healing energy. Many lay there and feel nothing in their body as I work on them. Some tell me they can feel a tingling through their body, while others report feeling something suddenly being lifted from their body as I snap something away, or perhaps we could say with Hippocrates, "pull and draw away some diverse impurity"

But here we had one who was quite unbelievably different. While I was running my hands over an area of the body where there was no problem he would lay there quite motionless. But then I found to my surprise that the moment my hand entered the area where there was negative energy and I could feel the resistance against my hand, his body would begin to jump uncontrollably. We soon found it was necessary for his wife or whoever had driven down to my home with him, to hold his legs in order to stop them from suddenly jumping up and falling over the side of the couch. I had experienced dramatic reaction to the healing energy on a few other patients, but as you will soon discover, this one went a little further than any of the others who had reacted in this particular way. Mind you, this visible and uncontrollable reaction is quite a normal thing with animals but only seems to happen with a small number of humans.

This patient has made the trip to my home a number of times, feeling that each time he had a healing session with me he gained a little more strength and comfort. This was borne out one day when I saw his car arrive in my drive, but instead of seeing his helpers unfold his wheelchair for him, they lifted one of those walkers with two little wheels from the boot and he walked into my house in that fashion. Just two or three visits later, it was a very proud and happy man who walked up the path, up the two or three steps at the front door and into my hall with the aid of no more than an ordinary walking stick. At this stage there were still one or two places where the negative energy had refused to leave, and each time my hand reached one of them, his body would jerk as if he was being given an electric shock.

About this time he rang me from his home and told me he would not be able to keep his appointment for the next day as he had transport problems and would ring me again next week for a new one. Then as an after thought he said "Do you think you could give me what you call absent healing if you have some spare time?" I assured him I would do that, but did not know when it might be. However, at 10 am next morning I did find some spare time, and walked into my healing room with a view to asking him to be placed on the couch to allow me to work on him. As I stepped up to the couch, I glanced at the clock on the other side of the room, and noticed it was showing exactly 10 am. I worked on him until I could feel no more pressure against my hand over any part of the couch, then walked away to carry on with some other duties I needed to do. Soon after this my phone rang and I picked it up to find that on the other end of the line was the one I had not long finished working on.

I was a little surprised to hear his voice but thought maybe he had solved his transport problems and wanted to come down after all. But that was not what he was ringing for at all. Far from it. He said "You started to work on me at 10 am this morning". I was just a little taken aback at this statement as I knew that no one could have told him that. I assured him I had done exactly that, then asked him how he could have known. His answer to that question proved to be one of the most interesting conversations I had heard in some time. He simply said "Well I was sitting in a chair here and all of a sudden my legs began to jump and I had trouble staying in the chair. I knew there was nothing else that had ever made my body react like that, so I felt sure you must have been working on me".

A few weeks ago this man and his wife made another trip to my home. He walked in with just a walking stick and came up the steps and into the healing room with no need for any other assistance. These two are always cheery enough people at any time, but on this occasion they both appeared to have an extra bit of a smile on their faces. Sensing that some thing was different, I asked them what was so amusing. They both laughed a little, and then the husband said, "We were just thinking how we would have loved to have you with us a few days ago. As you know, it is now more than a year since my cancer specialist gave me one year to live, so we thought we would pay him a visit and let him see the progress I have made".

Apparently, they had walked in to his surgery and he had appeared to be a little shocked to see his patient who was supposed to be with the angels by now, getting along with no more assistance than a walking stick. He said to them "My word you are not in your wheelchair". His patient then went on to tell him why, giving him some details concerning his visits to my healing room. At this stage I asked him whether they had been game enough to tell the oncologist about the way his body always jumps when my hand comes up against the negative energy. His simple reply was to tell me that was the funny bit that they were smiling about and it was also the reason why they would have liked me to have been present just to see the strange look on their oncologists face when he mentioned that.

Then I said to him, "I'll bet you didn't mention the absent healing I gave you while you were in Auckland with your body nearly jumping out of the chair?" At this stage, they both laughed and told me that was the bit they would really have loved for me to have had the pleasure of experiencing. He said when they left they had the impression he really thought that the cancer may not be affecting his spine too badly now, but surely it must be affecting his brain instead if he really believes like that. Oh well, I don't know what age his oncologist was, but as they say, he won't learn any younger, and it is never too late to learn.

Like I said early in this chapter, I know it works but don't press me for too much detail on how it works, it really only matters that it does.

How much more proof do the sceptics with closed minds want before they accept that there are more things in Heaven and Earth than they have yet dreamed of. How long will they continue to ignore the overwhelming amount of evidence which should prove to them without a shadow of a doubt, not only that Magnetic Healing really does work, but that it will also work with the patient many miles away.

A letter received from another grateful patient I had given absent healing to surely says it all.

"Dear Mr Lambert, I would like to thank you for absent healing my body. I know when you carried out some healing. I was standing by my kitchen table preparing our evening meal when I felt a sudden ping behind my left knee. It was of such sharpness and intensity that I looked down expecting to see a spurt of blood shooting out.

My old workhorse of a body has had many aches and pains, and I am very grateful and surprised that I find many things have disappeared. I no longer have to go to the toilet several times during the night, which means I am sleeping better. My tummy is no longer bloated, and I can walk easily on my left leg, as the pain in my foot has gone. God bless you". E. S.

So much for the sceptics. When will they ever learn. Isn't it a strange coincidence that these things always just happen to take place at the same time I am working on that person from some distant place.

A little earlier I mentioned a book titled "Radionics". A few words from the author David Tansley may give us a good clue as to what is going on in such cases as the above. He says, "that the search for the cause of disease must extend beyond the purely physical into the realisation that each individual exists not in a state of isolation, but is swimming in an immense sea of energy, of which he or she is an integral part, and in so being is a part of his or her fellow beings". My word David, you really hit the nail firmly on the head with that statement didn't you. Actually it is something I could have written myself as I have made a statement so close to that many times to groups of people at meetings wherever I have been. But the reason I wanted to quote from David's wonderful little book was mainly to show you that many minds are being tuned to precisely the same level of knowledge and understanding even though they may be living many miles apart and have never had the pleasure of meeting. While they may not have met in the physical, it became obvious that they are meeting on a mind level by tuning to the same frequency of vibration at which a particular truth vibrates and becomes reality to them. As far back as the 1930's Dr Ruth Drown of California reasoned that we all live in a vast field of energy that surrounds the planet, and that we are in effect all connected by this field.

The use of this sea of energy is nothing new. Rather its use is gradually being restored as more and more people open their minds to the truth of its existence. Healers have exercised this function in all ages. Surely it is enough for us to know that cures have taken place. But does it matter if we do not fully understand in what manner, or by what agency. This must be of less consequence than the fact itself. Undoubtably the law which governed them in all former ages is the same law which operates today, universal in its operation and eternal in duration.

When the Centurion approached Jesus and asked him to come quickly lest his servant should die, he was well aware that the distance between him and the ailing servant did not really exist. He knew and understood perfectly well, that all he needed to do was to raise his hand and say to the Centurion "Go home, thy servant liveth". Oh yes, if we can just have the "faith that moves mountains" and know that even as you ask, so will you receive, then we too, as he said can do the things which he did. They are not miracles in the sense that we in our ignorance think of miracles. We tend to consider a miracle as something which for us is the untouchable, the unobtainable. And of course we are right, as long as we believe that. You are what you believe, and nothing more and nothing less than exactly that.

When we can cast out the doubts and the fears, and know that there are no limits to our abilities except those which we place there with our negative thoughts then we can perform these things which we formally thought of as being miracles. Continue to believe as our so called scientists appear to do, that if you can not understand how it works, it doesn't, then you will stagnate in your thinking and in your beliefs as they do. These things may be "well outside the traditional boundaries of science" as we know it, but science needs to widen their limits, if they must insist on having any limits at all.

I well remember the day a Chinese doctor who was suffering from severe headaches asked me if I would attempt to find the problem and to do whatever I could to relieve it. I worked very hard on him for some time, spending most of the time around the head. After I had finished and sat back to relax he made what was for me, a very interesting statement He said "Colin, I can understand what you are doing when you work like that, but I am also well aware why most doctors would have no idea what it was all about. I spent several years learning to be a doctor and in all that time I hardly ever remember the word 'Energy' mentioned. But since then, I have also trained as an acupuncturist, and during that training energy was the word I probably heard more often than any other. We were told about chakras, meridians, and energy flow through the body. We learned that when a group of cells has become, as you put it, out of phase, this means there is a blockage acting like a dam, which is holding back the flow of energy to that particular group of cells. We were then shown how to use needles to break down the blockage to allow the energy to flow through freely to restore those cells to normality and to allow the body to return to it's normal state of health. But what amazes me about the way you work, is that you are doing exactly that, but without needles. Just using your hands to get that vital energy force moving again."

I have often thought about that statement over the years since I first heard it. After all it came from a medical doctor, but one with the added wisdom of a trained acupuncturist. I felt it answered a lot of questions for me. It made it just that much easier for me to understand why I had been having so much trouble attempting to get through the barriers which most medical people seemed to place around themselves the moment I mentioned the fact that I was working with energy. Perhaps it had not quite occurred to me before that I was almost speaking a foreign language to them. How could I have imagined that one who had spent 6 or 7 years learning how to help people who were ill would not even have been given basic training concerning the most important part of man, the ebbing and flowing of the lifeforce throughout the body. That which gives it life, and without which the dying cells would soon bring about the demise of the whole body if the condition was allowed to proliferate.

Just think about all of those electrical goods sitting in your home. These days nearly everyone has items such as a heater, a fan, a stove, a radio and a television among others. But what do you have when there is a power break which has stopped their life force from flowing through them. Nothing more than a collection of useless articles cluttering up your home. There is no heat coming from your heater, no sound from your radio or television. They are for all intents and purposes dead, when their life force has been blocked. And we are not that much different to them in that respect. Cut off your connection to the universal lifeforce energy, and like that radio or television there will be no sound coming from us either.

This is what happens when our link with this energy has been totally severed, similar to pulling out the plug on any one of those machines just mentioned. But suppose you are watching your favourite television programme, when suddenly you loose the sound. You have a picture, but nothing comes from the speaker. Somewhere in there you have a fault, the electrical energy is still reaching a large portion of the many different parts which go to make up that instrument. It is not dead. Its lifeforce has merely been blocked from flowing through to one of the many parts which go to make up the whole instrument.

If you bring that analogy over to your healing couch where a patient is laying, be it in the physical or the etheric counterpart, you now have in front of you an instrument, namely a body, which like your television is still connected to the lifeforce which animates it and makes it capable of what we may refer to as existence. The 'silver cord' as the Bible refers to this connection has not been severed, but somewhere in that physical body there has been a malfunction, so like your television, one part of it is not operating as it was designed to do. Perhaps it is a kidney which has had its line of communication with the rest of the body blocked. The lifeforce no longer flows into that part of the body and so we have what we may refer to as a sick kidney.

This is where the acupuncturist would work to break down the dam which is blocking the flow of life giving energy to that particular organ, and of course, as our Chinese doctor was intimating, this is also the area where the magnetic healer would apply the energy in order to restore the flow to that group of cells known as a kidney. But again I say that if there is anything wrong with what I have called magnetic healing then it is the fact that it is far too simple. When you come up against that particular place over the body where your hand would no longer move any further you are well aware that beneath it is an area where the lifeforce is not reaching. You know there is a group of cells right there which are dying due to the lack of life giving energy which is needed to allow them to work properly.

But the vital question here is, do you happen to know the name that has been given to this particular group of cells? In other words do you know exactly where to find the kidney? And this is where the doctor and energy healer part company. When a very angry doctor tells me in no uncertain terms that he could not believe I could possibly do anything for anyone when I didn't know where the organs were and he has spent 6 or 7 years learning about them, I am well aware that I would be wasting my breath if I was to tell him that was of no consequence. All the healer needs to know is where that blockage is which is stopping the lifeforce from reaching the organ. Break that down, and the organ, now being fed once again will restore itself and begin functioning as it was meant to do. If the doctor watching me tells me when I have finished that the group of cells I have just been working on is called a kidney, then so be it, but whether I know the name which has been given to that group of cells has no bearing on whether the patient's body will be restored to normality or not.

When you have called the etheric counterpart of your patient onto the couch in front of you, you visualise where the feet are and begin your work from there. You can tell when your hand reaches the torso by the much wider area you have to work on compared to when your hand was following a much narrower leg. So this gives you a fair idea of what part of the body you are working on. But whether the place your hand has suddenly been stopped at is over the kidney or the pancreas is much more difficult to determine. So it is just as well that there is no need whatsoever to know which organ you are working on. Only to be aware that this is the area where a group of cells have become out of phase due to the lack of lifeforce and needs to be restored.

You may not discover until some time later which organ you were working on. Very often I am not certain of this until I receive a letter or a phone call from the patient to inform me her pancreas, her kidney or what ever is now working properly again. I appear to have rambled on a bit about this, but strange to say, I have to do that for the sake of those who find it almost impossible to understand something so simple. If I was trying to get through to these ones something much more complicated, then I probably could have explained it in a lot less words, and they would have nodded their head and said "Yes, I can see that alright". But when they KNOW that nothing could be as simple as that, then it takes a lot more explanation. I have been reading some interesting information concerning a Dr Cornelia Featherstone. She is a medical doctor who trained in Germany. In recent years she has been living and working at Findhorn, the famous and long established alternative community in Scotland and has evolved a practice that incorporates complementary and orthodox healthcare. She points out that the British Medical Association has gone so far as to recommend that doctors acquaint themselves with local providers of non-conventional therapies.

Dr Featherstone says she is fascinated with the complementary modalities that use energy as part of their therapy. This is a very exciting area and we are finding out more and more about energy and health. At present it is as if the various 'energy based' therapies are mountain peaks sticking up out of the fog. The peaks we can see we understand, but as yet the valleys between them are full of fog, and there is so much which is not understood. She recommends that complementary practitioners spark a relationship with the general practitioners in their area and tell them about what they do. What a wonderful idea Dr Featherstone. I can go along with that 100%. But it would appear there is one small problem that you do not seem to be aware of. It may be the fact that because your "parachute" is wide open and your are prepared to listen to alternative practitioners, you have not realised that you are still very much in the minority as far as orthodox medical people are concerned. The story I told concerning the Dr who chased me from his hospital because he considered I had just gone there to waste his time, is just one of many I could mention. Right here in my home town I had to visit my doctor for a check-up before I could have my driver's licence renewed. Before leaving I suggested that perhaps if he had some spare time one day he would like to give me a ring as there were a number of things concerning my healing work which I thought may be of interest to him. His reply was short and to the point "You'll be lucky". Of course, needless to say, I wasn't lucky as I haven't heard from him.

Reaching out your hands to one in need with a view to allowing your body to be used as a channel for the universal loveforce is a privilege which should not be taken lightly. Whether you have the physical body on a couch or table in front of you, or whether you are visualising that one laying there, even though he or she may be 10,000 miles away your responsibility is the same. You must take the work seriously and treat it in every way with the boundless respect it deserves. You must learn to be a good listener because many times you will find a patient has come to you in a very upset and disturbed condition, and as much as anything else they are looking for someone who will let them unburden themselves of what appears to them to be an overwhelming level of stress which seems to be threatening to destroy them. More often than not these will be of the feminine gender, and may well be overloaded by the responsibilities of running a home with several children, or maybe it is because they have a husband or partner who they have found they cannot confide in concerning their problems. I have lost count of the number of times one such as this has suddenly burst into tears on my couch or cried her eyes out on my shoulder. Healers are for leaning on when someone finds their burden is such that they are finding it difficult to stand tall on their own two feet.

But many times, after having told that one to just let it all go and put all that pent up bitterness and distress behind them they walk out my door feeling 10 feet tall. Most of these have already visited the doctors surgery but have found that walking out the door grasping a piece of paper for a prescription for another bottle of tranquillisers was of little help and the burden just became that little bit heavier. This is one of the reasons why I prefer to have the patient on the couch in the physical form if possible but that does not mean to say that working absently on one such as this will be of no assistance. There are usually physical problems as well as mental in these cases, so if you restore a malfunctioning liver which is dragging the patient down in health then she is better able to cope with other levels of unease.

Whichever way you work just do your best. Put your heart and soul into it and know that in doing this work you are never alone. Ask and you will receive, and the patient will receive with you. Perhaps we should bring this chapter to a close at this point and set off on a very different path in more ways than one.

8. ENGLAND – CROP CIRCLE COUNTRY

I have already mentioned travelling to Australia, Canada and the United States to lecture and to teach but as I said at the end of the last chapter we now set off on a different path. Different in two respects. One is because we will be going to none of those places I have mentioned, but about as far as it is possible to go from New Zealand in England and Wales. The other way in which this chapter will be different will be recording my experience in that country in search of what have been commonly called 'Crop Circles'. You may well be wondering why I am about to write something such as this in a book which is supposed to be about magnetic healing.

I do not blame you at all for thinking that because for many I realise there would appear to be no possible connection. For those who have already read any one of my first four books my reason for doing so would be better understood, but for those of you who have not done so, may I ask you to simply read on and hopefully by the time you read the end of this chapter, you too will discover the connection which may well be eluding you at this moment. When my first book "WHY" was published in London in 1970 I received several letters from readers who wanted to tell me how much they had enjoyed reading about the healing work and some of the things I had mentioned such as the hypnosis I was doing at that time, but were at a loss to understand why I had included such things as UFO's etc. Hopefully in this chapter I will be able to answer any queries in that respect.

I see the universe as nothing more than energy. Energy in it's many forms and frequencies of vibration. The little Maori girl who watched me remove cancer from her mother and then declared on the way home in the car that she would rather go to that doctor than the other ones because she had not seen the other doctors take a lump of black meat from her mummy's tummy and throw it away in the corner of the room, was not psychic as many people would suggest. For me the simple explanation is that this child was able to see atoms vibrating at a higher frequency than most other people.

The doctor who asked me who the dark man was standing beside me while I was giving healing to his wife, plus a lady he saw just standing behind me watching the proceedings, was not a man who is so crazy that he should not be practicing as a doctor at all. This sort of thinking which so many people, and particularly the scientific and the very religious still cling to, does no more for them than show their ignorance of what matter is really all about. I sometimes describe what we call solid matter as frozen energy. Surely every atom is a mass of whirling energy and what else goes to make up everything other than what has been termed "the building blocks of nature" the atoms.

Everything we see with our physical eyes we only see because these particular items are made up of atoms vibrating at a slow enough rate for our very slow eye-brain combination to perceive. After all, we do not really see with our eyes. I see them as being intermediary between the object we are perceiving and the brain which is registering our recognition of that object. Speed up the movement of that object such as a rapidly spinning propeller on an aeroplane and the brain no longer has enough time to register the fact that the eye has seen it before it has moved on, so we no longer see the solid object we call a propeller. But photograph it with a camera which has a very fast shutter and use fast film and you can prove that at a given fraction of a second that blade was in a certain position. I have a photo of a bomber taking off the ground. At the time this photo was taken the engines would have been on full throttle as it lifted away, yet not one of those propellers is moving in the photo. My Kirlian machine with which I photograph the energy surrounding a finger does not have any lens whatsoever. It works on a high frequency energy, and does not show the physical finger which is made up of atoms vibrating at a low enough frequency for you and I to see, but only makes visible the rapidly vibrating atoms which go to make up what we commonly refer to as the aura or lifeforce which animates and gives life to the physical being.

Yes I know, I said we would be going to England in this chapter and we are, but before doing so I am attempting to help you to understand some of the reasons why it is so necessary if we are going to use energy to help people, to begin by understanding something about this thing we are using. When a healer is working over a body to remove a problem such as a cancer growth, then what I visualise taking place here is simply the energy you are applying to the body is speeding up the vibratory rate of the unwanted atoms and drawing them up through a so called solid body where they can be picked up in the form of what our little girl referred to as a lump of black meat and taken away out of the aura of the patient. And remember your body is not solid matter. It is atoms with spaces in between like all other matter, infinitesimal as those spaces may be. During my years of study I have come to realise that all of the phenomena such as those things which we refer to as UFO's, Crop Circles, mutilated animals etc, are all the product of people who have long come to understand the true nature of energy with the result that they can use it and manipulate it in such a way that we have not even dreamed of. Hence my intense interest in what I can learn from the actions of those who already have the knowledge.

If we as a race were to open our eyes and our minds to what has been going on around us for so long instead of keeping them so closed as we have been doing we would discover a whole new science for us to use to change our world into something of which as yet we have barely dared to dream. Gone would be this negative low frequency thing we call "science", to be superseded by the science of the higher frequency energies which we in our ignorance refer to as miracles. In Chapter 3 I mentioned a small book with the title "Handbook of Magnetic Cure" and quoted briefly from it. There is one more small quote from that book I would like to add here. "We do not regard any cure as a miracle but as the result of a fixed law of nature, the successful employment of magnetic power being no more marvellous or supernatural than similar events daily taking place among us now. You all hold within your grasp all the remedial agents that you have need of, but you do not know how to use them. That all powerful force that we call magnetism has within itself the power to harmonise all the forces of the human body to prevent disease. When disease or inharmony, which is the same, has found an abiding place in the physical form, magnetism has the power to eradicate it not only to subdue it, but to entirely overcome it. You are standing today on the threshold of this new science. It has always been with you, but because of its simplicity men and women have considered it to be of no account. But the time is fast coming when you will understand what disease is, and what is its remedy."

My word, how often have I said to so many people the only thing that I know of that is wrong with magnetic healing is the fact that it is too simple and highly educated people know that nothing could be that simple.

Having said all this perhaps it is time for us to think about climbing aboard that big bird again and taking ourselves off to the other side of planet earth to see what we can find in our search for an understanding of the endless uses of energy. A man came to my home with a friend and his wife who were visiting from Bristol in England. While giving them some healing I mentioned that I hoped to travel to his country in the not too distant future to do two things. One would be to lecture and to teach my healing techniques to anyone who would be interesting in learning them, and the other was to catch up on some of the things I have read about in that country, but had not had the pleasure of seeing. I told them this would include such things as ancient stone circles, and if I could visit at the appropriate time of the year, Crop Circles. The husband assured me he knew groups of people in different areas who would be interested in my work and his wife agreed they would be very happy to have me stay with them in their home if this should eventuate. A number of letters and a few phone calls later, a trip up to Shrewsbury and possibly London was arranged, and I set off across the world once again. Although I had been to England once before in 1979 when I took my wife up to Shetland Islands to meet some of her relatives, her father having migrated from there many years ago, I had not had the opportunity to visit the ancient sites at that time other than taking a bus trip from London out to Stonehenge and of course Crop Circles were something that had not yet arrived on the scene at all.

And so it was with some degree of apprehension that I set out on a voyage of discovery which was to be combined with my usual reason for such a trip, showing eager students how to become Magnetic Healers. What I was not aware of at this time was the fact that having already conducted so many very successful tours to several countries where almost all of my time and energy had gone into the latter of those two, the one who goes before me had arranged that this time my priority would be guided towards the former. And so it was that I was given the opportunity to speak to a few groups of interested people and to leave behind me some of them very capable of carrying on my work in my absence.

The husband in this team I stayed with was an excellent diviner of water and energies in general having been to many peoples homes to help with problems such as water flowing under their house and creating health problems for their family. I soon discovered that the groups of people he had referred to in my home some months before, were not necessarily people who were particularly interested in healing or had the desire to become healers. They tended to be people who were more interested in divining as he was, and so it was not too surprising to find that instead of meeting people who wanted to become healers as I have been used to doing everywhere I go, those I did meet were for the most part unaware that running your hands through the energy field of one with a health problem was actually divining of a different kind. Just as the water or oil diviner picks up or senses a different frequency of energy set up by the existence of that water or oil below the surface of the earth, so the healer is using his hands, a pendulum or an aura meter to detect the different frequency of the patients aura where it has been disturbed by the unbalancing of a group of cells in a particular part of that body.

But I soon found that for most diviners, divining is something that you do when you are looking for water or oil as I have just mentioned, but the divining of that different frequency of vibration in a persons aura was something which did not come into the orbit of their thinking pattern at all. After meeting a few of them, I began to wonder what I was doing in England if this was to be the way in which my trip was to progress. Sometimes it can be very difficult when we suddenly find our preconceived ideas about something do not appear to be working in the way we had expected. This was especially true for me at this time because of all those other wonderful trips which had so obviously been under the control of a guiding hand, and had always been shown to have the teaching of others to become healers as the focal point of the whole operation.

And now here I was, 12,000 miles from home and stuck with a group of people who appeared to have little interest in the very things I had travelled all that way to speak about. There had to be some other purpose behind all this and indeed there was, but at that stage I had not yet found it. My friend did bring about six people to his home one evening, but although there was some interest shown in my work, it was a long way from the sort of ecstatic enthusiasm I had become used to almost everywhere I went.

My friend had told me he would be happy to drive me around anywhere in his area to look at anything which I was particularly interested to see, and in this he was even better than his word. One day was spent seeing the sights at Avesbury in Wiltshire. This massive embankment and ditch which make up Avesbury Henge is part of a 5,000 year old 28 acre site with a large megalithic stone circle and two smaller circles of stone. Silbury Hill, Europe's largest megalithic structure is not far away and can be seen from the circle. For me there was something about the energy in this area which seemed to be saying, 'now perhaps you are beginning to understand why you are in England'. We were carrying a set each of those L wires I have previously mentioned and as we approached a huge standing stone many feet high, my friend who had been here several times before and had spent a lot of time measuring the energy fields in the area, told me to stand back a few yards from the stone and hold my two wires in my hand with the long ends pointing towards it. He told me he had measured this particular stone before and had found there was eight different levels of energy coming from it between the ground and the top. I found it hard to believe how this could be, but my doubts were soon shattered. He told me to look at the base of the stone while holding the wires and to ask to be shown where level seven of this energy was coming from. He then said to slowly bring my eyes up the stone as I made this request. By the time my gaze had reached about three-quarters of the way up, I was beginning to think he must be having me on as nothing whatsoever was happening. Then just as I was feeling sure this had to be a waste of time the wires slowly parted and pointed to my left and right instead of straight at the stone as they had been doing.

Of course, eight different levels of energy from the ground up he had said. So where should I have expected to find the seventh level? No other place than 7/8 of the way up of course, and that was exactly where the wires parted as my gaze reached that area. By this time I was finally beginning to consider that maybe after so many overseas trips where I had spent almost all of my time and energy showing others how to use energy, this was one occasion where the reverse situation would exist. Perhaps it was my turn to be shown a few new facts concerning this energy in its many forms and frequencies of vibration which I had been telling others about for so long. As you will see before we leave England, this assumption turned out to be true in more ways than one.

That day was a long and tiring one, so the following day we reckoned it was time for a rest, and that was how we spent it. But the next day we were on the road again. This time we visited Glastonbury and then went on to Stonehenge. As we had both visited Stonehenge before we did not spend a lot of time there, but were more interested in trying to find a large Crop Circle which we had been told was not far away. We finally managed to find someone who told us to drive to the next road which ran behind Stonehenge but still within sight of it. This proved to be a beautiful very large and complicated Pictogram consisting of many circles of varying sizes. Unfortunately it was about a month old and as the bending of the wheat does not stop it from growing, it had grown up enough to spoil what must have been an incredible sight when it was first discovered. Its age however, did not exclude it from containing much of the energy which was used to make it. In fact, when we could not see it from the road, we soon pinpointed the direction in which to cross the large field by using our L wires as diagnostic tools.

From here we drove quite a long distance to Badbury castle where we discovered another interesting, but once again quite old Pictogram of an entirely different shape.

It was interesting to walk into one of those massive patterns in wheat, some of them two or three hundred feet across and to speculate on the source of the energy which had been used to make them. A little later we will be taking a very close look at that particular mystery, if you wish to call it that, but before we do I would like to make mention of a little trip we did across the country into Wales. My friend told me we would be driving through to Swanson where we would be meeting an old friend of his. He owned a factory there, and also a Holiday Camp where he would provide us with a place to stay.

All this sounded great, particularly as he assured me that a workshop had been arranged for me the day after we arrived and it would be held in quite a large room at the factory. They were apparently expecting a good attendance, so I was pleased with the thought that at least I would be spending some time doing what I felt I had travelled halfway around the world to do. By the time we arrived at the Holiday camp in Swanson, it was late in the afternoon and we barely had time to settle in and very little time to do anything about eating before our host informed us he would be picking us up and driving us out to a large house in the country where there was a meeting being held. He said he did not know a lot about the speaker but thought he was from Australia and did some form of healing.

This all sounded interesting, so it was with some anticipation that we arrived at the house and were ushered into a very large room where there were at least 30 or more people already gathered. We managed to find a place to sit down in a very big bay window which had a seat around it and we made ourselves as comfortable as possible. There was very little light in the room but in a corner at the far end I could just make out the unmistakable shape of a healing couch. When everybody was settled down, a man came in from a back room and stood behind it just as I would have done if this had been one of my meetings. I remember thinking how much he looked like a man I taught Magnetic Healing several years ago, but of course dismissed any such possibility as this was Wales, not Auckland, New Zealand, where that man lived when he came to one of my workshops.

But as he began to speak and his voice sounded even more familiar, than his looks, I could not help turning to my friends and whispering to them something like "What are they trying to do to me, I have travelled half way

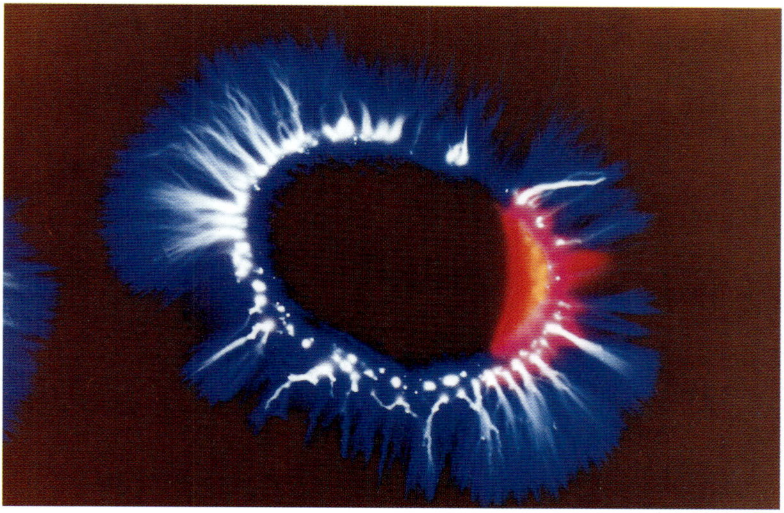
kirilan photo of fingertip

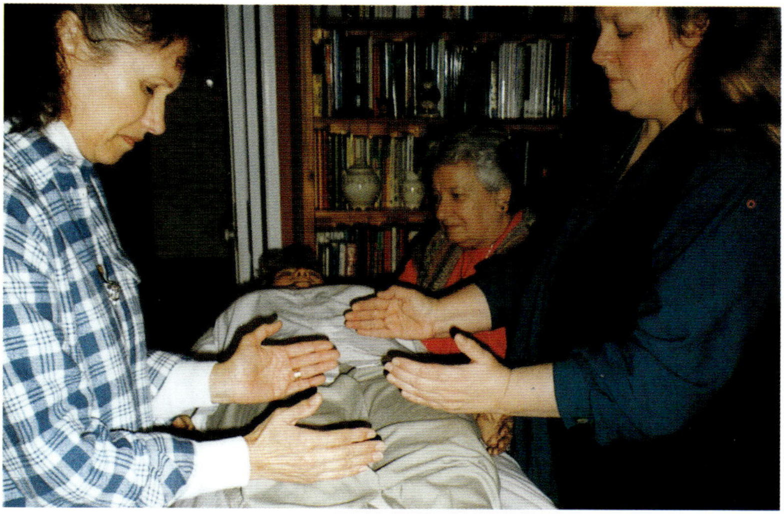
Healing session at Nowra, Australia

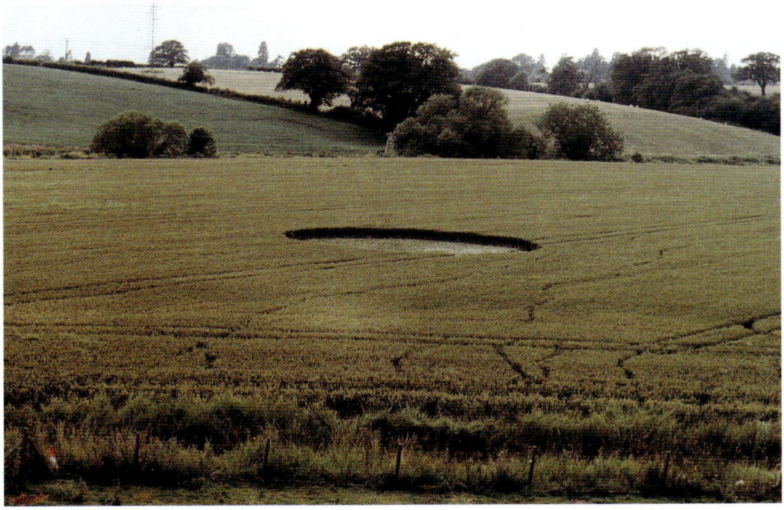

Shrewsbury crop circle from bridge

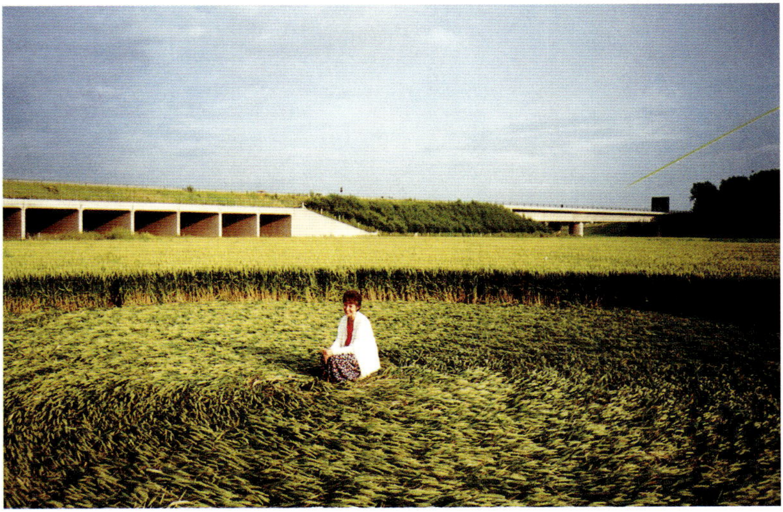

Shrewsbury crop circle close up

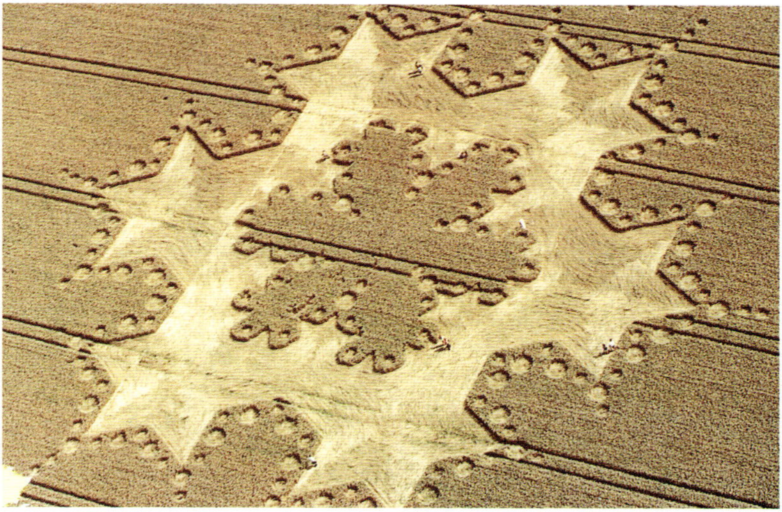

Crop circle at Milk Hill.

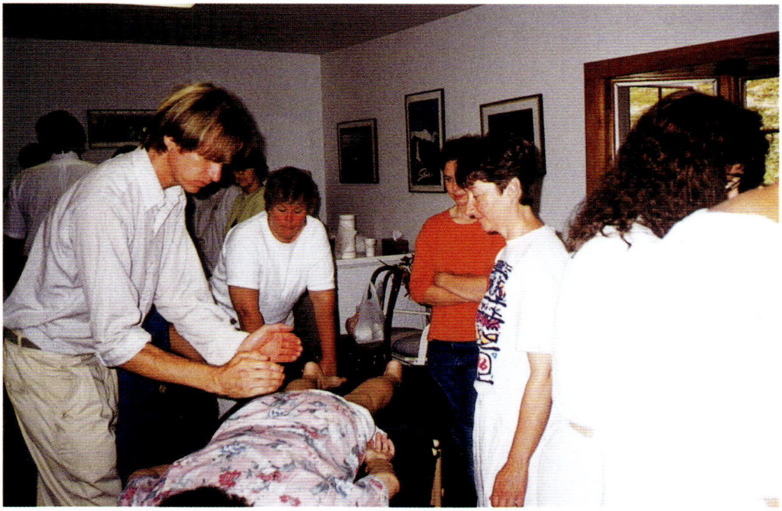

Students practising at Lisa's home in Vermont.

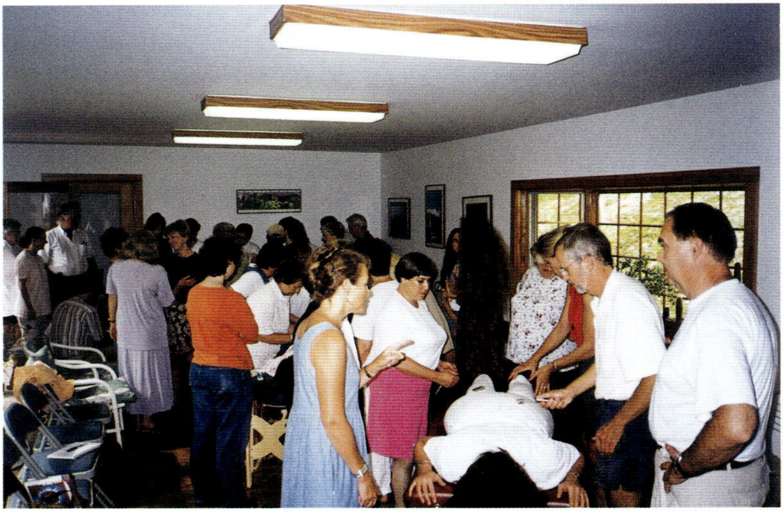

50 students from two previous days gather to practise.

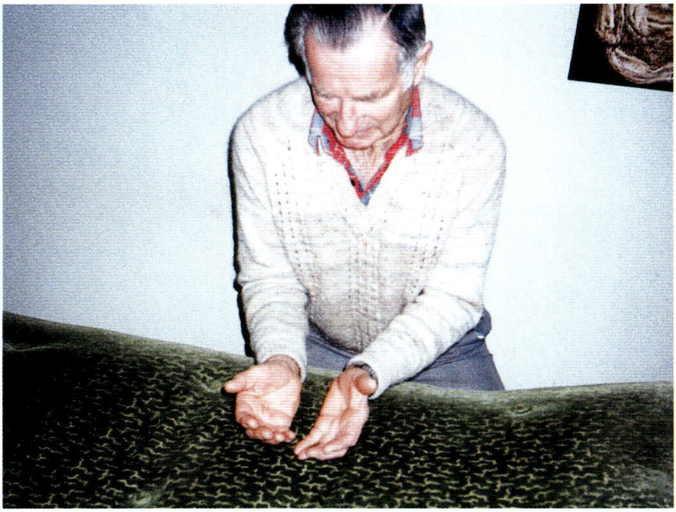

Cupping the negative energy away.

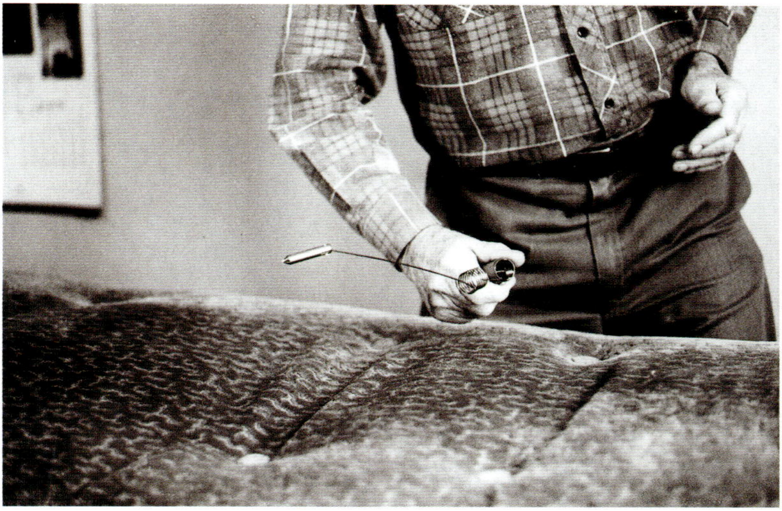

Measuring the negative energy. Absent healing

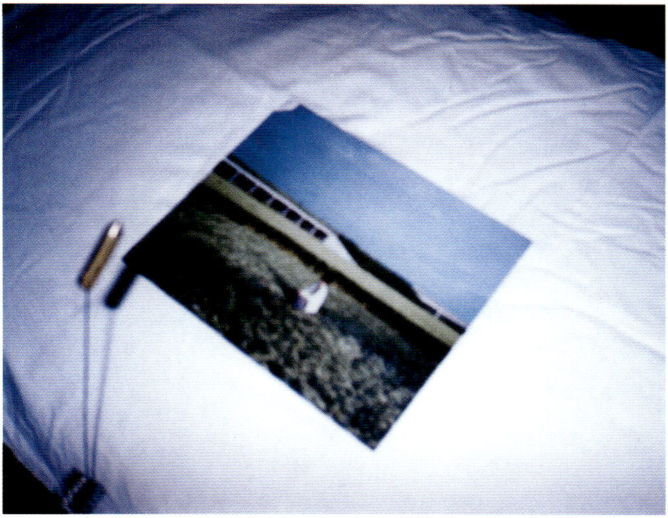

Measuring the energy above photo of Shrewsbury crop circle

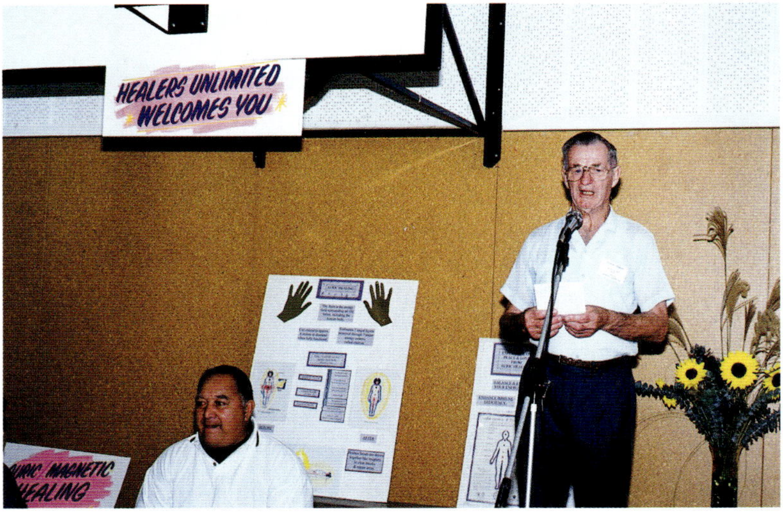

Speaking to public gathering at "Healers Unlimited" meeting. Palmerston North. April 99

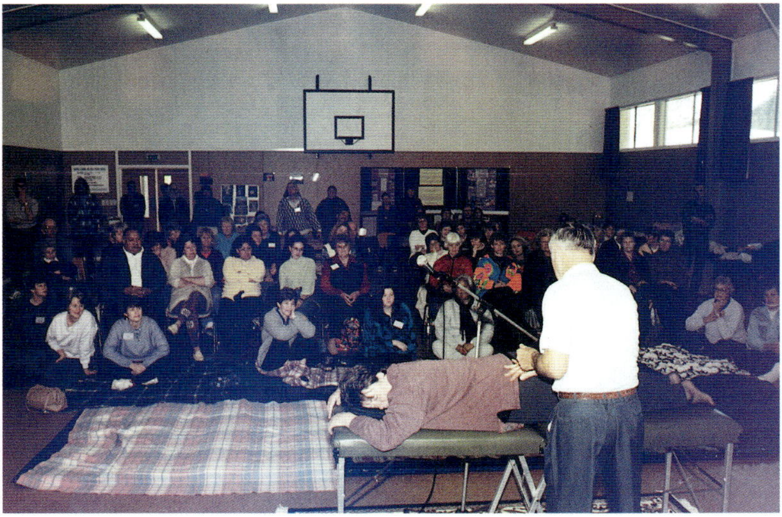
Demonstrating Magnetic Healing. Palmerston North

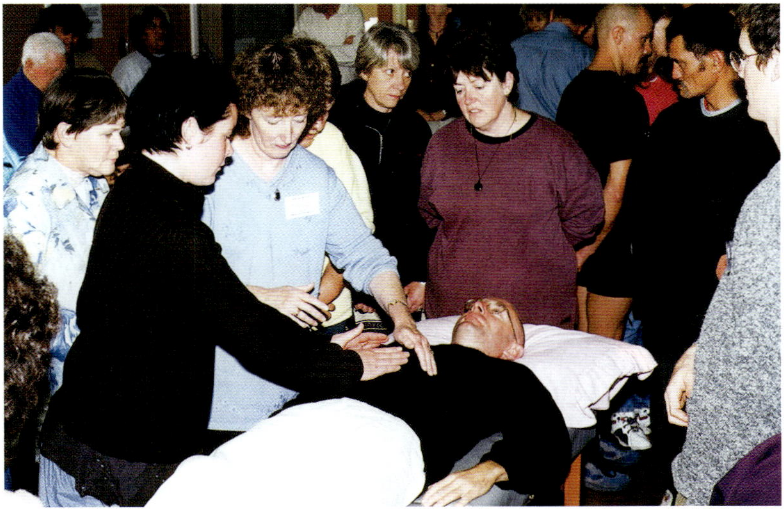

Students giving healing. Palmerston North. Kathy, organiser in blue.

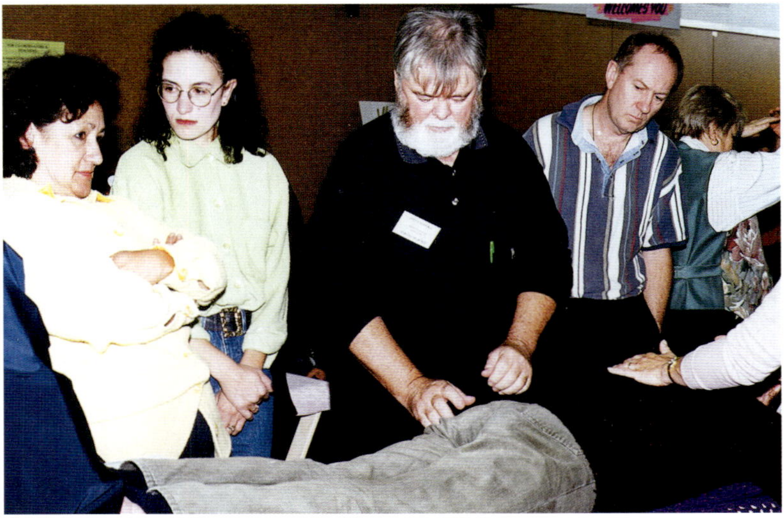

The "Sceptic" shows his skills. Palmerston North.

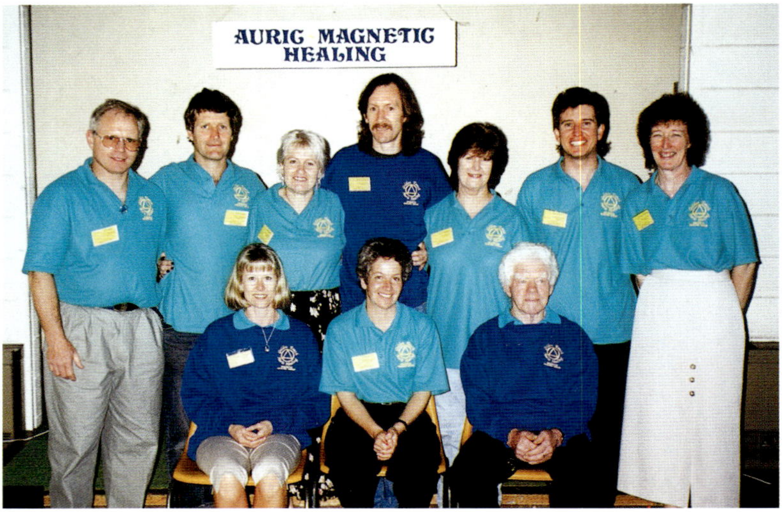

Kathy's Magnetic Healing Group. Palmerston North

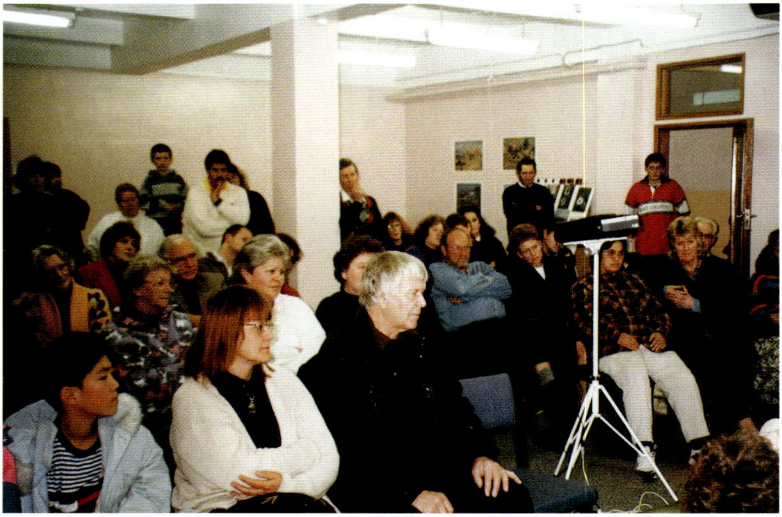
Public Meeting. Wanganui. 60 present. Note the intense concentration of the audience as they watch a demonstration of Magnetic Healing.

around the world, then way out into the country to listen to someone talking about the healing I had shown him how to do back home in New Zealand". And when I say what are 'they doing to me', I don't mean my two friends who had driven me there, I mean my friends and helpers upstairs. Was this supposed to be some sort of joke, or were they trying to teach me sort of lesson.

But worse was to come. We had only arrived that afternoon but apparently my ex pupil had been in the area for a few days, and we heard his organisers reminding the people gathered about the teaching class the speaker would be holding tomorrow at about the same time as mine was to be held. Needless to say, as his class had been advertised for some time and his presence in the area had already attracted a lot of attention, most of the people who would be interested in what he would be showing them were already booked to attend his workshop and were only being reminded of the time and place.

Disaster was about the only word I could think of to cover such an unbelievable set of coincidences, but then I remembered how many times I had told people that in my life there are no coincidences, whatever happens is all a very necessary part of a plan. Like everybody else, I am still learning, and if this was the lesson which they wanted me to learn at this particular time as I walk the path of the school of life, then perhaps at least a part of that lesson was to be able to accept gracefully what appeared to be on the surface a let down after all the time and energy I had spent since I left New Zealand just getting to a city in Wales so that I could pass on my knowledge and experience to whoever wanted to listen and to learn. It was a little difficult not to feel a bit hurt by all this, but I know the more hurt I felt by all this, the less I would learn from the lesson of humility. I was obviously being taught that night. So the only thing to do as we left the room about two hours later was to go up to the couch and shake the speakers hand. I am not sure now which of us was the most surprised to realise that in this one room in a country area of Wales were two New Zealanders drawn together under most unusual circumstances.

We did have a small but very attentive and interested group at our little workshop the next morning, but it was difficult to stop my mind from thinking now and then about my ex student just down the road with his room full of people gathered together to learn from him. Such is the way in which we learn to grow as we walk the path of life in order to learn the lessons we came here to learn. Humility, thankfulness for every blessing which comes our way, and the strength to carry on with that which we have come here to do. Even in the face of what may appear at the time to be an injustice. Learn your lessons well, and you will find that with each one mastered you have climbed another rung in that long ladder of evolvement which leads to the mountain top and a recognition of your oneness with all of creation and the divine creative force variously labelled God, Allah or whichever name you happen to be told you should call it.

A day or two after we arrived back in Bristol I had intended to book a bus trip to my next destination 100 or more miles to the north. This was Shrewsbury where a man I had met in New Zealand a few years earlier had offered to organise some meetings and to have me stay for a few days in their home. But my man in Bristol, not satisfied with having driven me to several areas to view stone circles and crop circles, plus a trip into Wales, decided he should also take me to Shrewsbury in his car. I meet some wonderful generous people as I travel through different countries and here again was one who was certainly no exception to that rule. We were warmly welcomed into Johns home when we arrived in Shrewsbury and my friend stayed the night with us before driving back home to Bristol the following day.

There was a small group of just 6 people for me to teach the following day, but as my notes say, small but very good. The lady whose home I worked in that day, was a medium and her friends were obviously very open minded with an awareness of the spiritual nature of man and all of this showed in their enthusiasm and their desire to learn all they could which may in some way help them to be able to serve humanity. We had a public meeting on the Friday evening, which in typical city style attracted a very small number of interested people.

But if I was looking for at least one day in England which would be one I would not forget in a long time the following day had to be the one. Early Sunday morning a lady had agreed to take me on the long drive to Heathrow Airport where I was booked with Air New Zealand for my flight home. Saturday afternoon was to be my last workshop and I felt sure that this time things would be a little more like normal. In spite of the small number at the public meeting on the previous evening I felt there had been enough interest there for at least several of them to attend the workshop next day and possibly, bring one or two of their friends with them.

As it turned out, that was an understatement. I think I have already mentioned that I do not like to have more than about twenty students at a workshop because it becomes too top heavy and it is difficult to find enough time in a three hour session to have each one come up beside me and show them how to feel the negative energy over the patients body and to remove some of it. For some reason it seems that no matter how may meetings I hold there are always those who will not arrive on time, so I usually find a 1 pm meeting rarely gets started before 1:15 as it is disturbing to have people still coming in the door after I have started. But on this occasion we already had 20 or more people sitting in rows in front of me eagerly waiting for me to begin.

I remember thinking how keen they must be to learn when for once we had them all here on time. But oh dear, it was not like that at all. There were still late comers and plenty of them. As the number crept up above the thirty mark and my organisers began running around looking for chairs they had never expected they would need, I began to wonder how I was ever going to manage a workshop of this size. They did finally stop coming through the door, but not until the number had reached more than forty, not to mention the panic level. However, I decided I would just have to talk for a little less time than I normally do, to allow more time for the students to come up and feel the energy. Fortunately we had a good patient, good that is from a point of view of the students. A good guinea pig as I sometimes refer to them has to be a bad one, otherwise it is not very long before there is nothing for the students to work on.

But this one had a serious enough problem for everyone to be able to feel the negative energy in one or other of the two or three places he had a problem. I was amazed at how well it went considering the large number of people I had to contend with. We did extend the length of that class quite a lot but I felt it was well worthwhile just to see so many very happy people finally leaving the meeting.

And was it really worth travelling all that way just for that? Well I will let you judge that for yourself but not until after you have read the contents of a letter I received from John my organiser and host some three months later.

"We are continuing with the healing training every other Thursday evening here in Shrewsbury at the same place you did your seminar. We meet from 7:00 pm to 10:30 pm and average about 20 people. Everyone seems to be really enjoying it."

That extract from his letter told me all I needed to know. My time had been well spent, and now in a city about as far away as it is possible to go from my home here in little Waihi, a town of 3,500 people in New Zealand, there are an ever increasing number of people with love in their hearts making the effort to give out some of that love to their fellow beings in need, by offering themselves to be used as channels for the healing energy.

I have mentioned early the next morning I was to be driven to Heathrow the London Airport to begin my journey home, so no doubt you will be saying to yourself, well that is the end of his English experience. But you would be very wrong if that was what you were thinking. Each night during the week I slept upstairs in that Shrewsbury home, I had laid in bed before going to sleep and put out a thought pattern onto the ethers in hope that someone out there might pick up my request and answer it. That request each night went something like this, "I have come halfway around the world for two good reasons. One was to show as many people as possible how they could be used as channels for the healing energy. For some reason this did not eventuate in anything like the way it has done in every other place I have been. I have been thinking that maybe I wasn't supposed to do a lot of work this time. Maybe the other reason I came here was more important for me on this trip. And yes, I have been lucky enough to visit some very interesting places and to learn more about energy. I have been able to walk onto some Crop Circles which I so desperately wanted to see. But they have all been at least a month old and lost much of their beauty. Would it not be possible for me to see a brand new one and to experience the power of its energy before I go home"

I was well aware that apart from the fact that there was very little time for this to happen, I also knew that Shrewsbury was not known as a Crop Circle area. I had already been to those areas. I had been to Stonehenge, one of those areas where energy abounds, not to mention the Avesbury circle and Silbury Hill where many of the best Pictograms have been discovered almost annually for several years now but not the day I was there. Was it really asking too much to expect one to be made in Shrewsbury just for my benefit? They do say, God loves a trier and he must love me. And why? Because when we finally arrived back at John's home about 5:30 there was two messages on his answer phone. One was for John, and would you believe the other was for Colin. It was a short message from the medium lady, whose home I had visited earlier in the week to do that small workshop. She said, "Will you tell Colin there is just a small piece in this evenings newspaper about a beautiful big crop circle which arrived last night. It is about a mile from your home and is just off the A5".

I could hardly believe what I was hearing. Only hours before I was to leave for home and about all I could think of saying was, 'thank you, thank you'. My friend rang a lady friend of his who he knew would be very interested and we agreed to meet her where the road, whose name I cannot remember met the A5, which runs down to Birmingham. When we arrived there we could see no sign of anything that looked remotely like a Crop Circle. Actually, we knew it could not be all that close as the news item had mentioned that it was in a field of wheat. There was no one in sight that we could ask for directions, nor were there any houses in view. Then I had an idea. I had bought two different items with me from John's home. One was my camera, and the other was a pair of the L wires I have already mentioned.

I took these out of the car and stood on the edge of the road holding them in front of me. I had no idea in which direction the Crop Circle may be. Only that it was somewhere close to the A5 and not far from the road on which we were standing at a point where it intersected with the A5. As I stood there with the two wires pointing away from me and held several inches apart, I said these words ' If this is a genuine Crop Circle and not a fake one, then I want to be shown where it is'. I slowly turned my body to the left hoping that at some point they would indicate to me the direction in which we must travel in order to find it. By the time I had pivoted around at 180 degrees. I was beginning to worry and wonder whether this was going to work as the wires moved slowly around with me and showed no sign of being disturbed in any way.

And then it happened. Suddenly my whole body stiffened, and the wires which I was holding several inches apart came together at the far end and pointed very precisely in one direction. I said to my friends that it had to be over in that direction, but they pointed out that there was no sign of any wheat there and to quite a large hill several hundred feet away. My answer to that was to tell them that it must be on the other side of the hill, particularly as the A5 ran right past this hill, so it would still be next to that highway as the newspaper had reported. So we took wires and camera and made our way down the highway where it skirted one side of the hill. By the time we reached the other side of that hill we could see the highway crossed quite a large bridge in front of us. This was a bridge which crossed the Severn River which runs right on down into Wales. When we were about half way across and already leaving the hill behind us, I noticed that on the other side of the bridge down below the level of the road where the river meandered its way in the direction of Wales, there was a large river flat completely covered in wheat.

And there, as you will see in the photo I took from the bridge, was a beautiful Crop Circle. (Page **122**) It was exactly that a Crop Circle. And not one of those fancy Pictograms which have manifested so many times now in several countries around the world and particularly in England. But nevertheless a beautiful sight. A fresh perfect circle, right out there in the middle of the field. Needless to say after taking that photo, we hurried down to inspect it. As we approached the circle I held my L wires out in front of me again, and right at the edge they suddenly split apart and pointed one to the left and one to the right indicating that there was a forcefield of some kind precisely at the outer edge. I then walked towards the centre and found that the moment I reached it the wires were drawn in again and crossed right over the centre.

So this was it. Now I felt I knew for certain my reason for my trip to England. To prove without a shadow of a doubt exactly what I had been telling people I had believed for a long time. Now I no longer needed to believe. Now I **KNEW.** And there is a world of difference between believing something and knowing it. Believing is something which you have been told such as the dogmatic beliefs of any particular religion. If you are bought up in a home where your parents belong to a religious faith and take you to church on Sunday and perhaps to Sunday school, then you will almost certainly grow up following in your parent's footsteps and having the same beliefs. But that is all they are. You cannot say that what you believe really is the whole truth and nothing but the truth, because you do not know. You may even get angry if someone argues with you and suggests that you do not have the truth. But remember your neighbour across the road goes to a different church, and their children have grown up with a completely different belief. Yet they are just as sure that their belief is the real truth as you are that yours is infallible.

Is it any wonder that religious beliefs have caused more wars and suffering, hatred and bitterness on this planet over many centuries than anything else. But let us look at my reasons for saying that I now knew instead of just believing. A few years ago I saw a documentary on our TV which had been made in England and sent out to Australia and New Zealand and probably other countries which I don't know about. It was a documentary which had been made to convince you, the viewer, that there was no mystery concerning Crop Circles and to assure you they were not made by little green men from Mars or whatever. And the way they "proved" this was to interview two men, Doug and Dave, who assured us they had made all the Crop Circles in England since they first appeared a few years earlier. They then went in to a field of corn and demonstrated how they had achieved this. They had a steel handle which they held, and on the other end of it there was a piece of wood which they kept pushing down with their foot in order to flatten the corn or wheat or whatever the Corp Circle had been made in.

One look at the finished product was enough for me as I already had seen some very good photos and some video tape which showed how neatly every stalk had been laid down side by side with not one out of place, where as the crop they had pushed down to the ground looked more like a very strong wind had flattened it. And now here in front of me was the positive proof. The corn in this particular circle had been laid in an anti clockwise direction, although many of them are clockwise. Every stalk was laying beside its neighbour and you can see from the photo on page 122 the stalks around the edge were standing straight and proud like sentinels with not one out of place. This would be very difficult to achieve with a piece of wood on a steel handle, particularly as it had arrived like all the others in the dark of night.

But even allowing for the remote possibility that somehow Doug and Dave, or any hoaxer for that matter had managed to achieve the seemingly impossible I knew for sure there was one thing they could have not brought about with that crude instrument, or for that matter, anything which has been invented as yet. Remember how I managed to find the circle. The best part of half a mile away my L wires pointed in the direction in which it was to be found. Even the hill in between did not stop them from picking up the energy which had been used to bend the wheat with in the first place. The same energy which split my wires apart as I approached the edge of that beautiful 67 foot circle, and then drew them in to cross each other at the centre.

There are some of the darker races on the planet who do not like you taking their photographs. They say you take something from them with the photograph. Maybe they know more than we think they do. You see I have discovered that every photo of a Crop Circle or Pictogram carries with it something of the energy which was used to create the circle in the first place. If I move my L wires towards the photo of our Crop Circle they will still cross over the centre just as they did over the real thing. And strange to say, this same law applies to a model of a pyramid if it has been built to the same specifications as the original Cheops. The photos on page 113 of my previous book "You Too Can Heal", show this phenomena very clearly.

As you can imagine it was a very happy man who returned to his hosts home a little later in the evening. I felt that my request having been granted in such an amazing way within hours of my departure time surely meant that the one who goes before me knew exactly what he was doing. This was what my trip to England had really been all about. Any teaching or healing on this trip was to be looked on as a bonus. I had already experienced plenty of other tours, and more were to come, where I had worked very hard with meetings and workshops crowding one another and little time to do any sightseeing or to rest and be a normal tourist for a while. I felt this was further borne out by the almost unbelievable story of my efforts to spend a few days in London lecturing and teaching. I did not want to go to London to see the sights as I had already done that in '79 with my wife. I wanted to go there to work. But it finally came home to me that this was not to be a part of the plan at all. There were no Crop Circles in London, but there would have been plenty of stress which I finally came to the conclusion my helpers did not want me to have in my 77th year.

Long before I left home I had spent quite a lot of time writing letters to 2 or 3 likely contacts I had been given as someone who may be interested in organising some meetings and maybe finding somewhere for me to stay for a few days. I have found that almost anywhere I travel around the world there is always plenty of people who are keen to offer me a bed and a meal in exchange for what they usually consider to be the privilege *(their word, not mine)* of having me in their home and maybe have me give some of their family healing in exchange, and to have the opportunity to pick up as much as they can from my many years as a healer. For this reason I found it difficult to understand why this was not happening in London. While I had no such problem in Bristol or Shrewsbury I was drawing a total blank in London.

I found it hard to believe when the thanks, but no thanks letters kept coming into my home and the bill for toll calls to London kept rising. Some of them referred me to some friend who they thought may be interested, but by the time I left New Zealand nothing had been arranged, so I allowed one week on my airline ticket with the thought that I could talk to these people more cheaply once I actually arrived in England. But my last desperate phone call from Shrewsbury to the lady who had finally agreed to organise something for me sounded like I would be heading for something not far short of a nightmare if I had continued on to London for the last week. She did not actually have any meetings arranged, but she did say she knew of a lady who would provide me with a bed for a few days. She said "You will have to pay something towards the meals, and as she works all day and does not own a car you will have to find your own way around. She will be there in the evening, but she will be away at work all day".

It sounded like it was about time for me to say "thanks, but no thanks" and in about as polite a way as possible, this is just about what I did. I did not mind helping towards the meals of course as I always like to do, but finding my way around London and no meetings actually organised, I reckoned that was a situation I could well do without. I rang Air New Zealand, and yes, they had a spare seat on this Sunday instead of the following one which I was booked on. At the time I did that, about mid-week, I was still disappointed that I had not had the opportunity to walk onto a nice new Crop Circle, and of course was not aware that someone up there had plans in motion which would see to it that this little piece of frustration would be swept away to be replaced by ecstatic satisfaction before I left the shores of England a few days later.

They do say, ask and thou shalt receive, and maybe we should learn that lesson a little better. It certainly worked for me, and I see no reason why it should not work for you if your motives for asking are not of a selfish nature. While there was of course a certain degree of self satisfaction having my request granted, I felt that it went much deeper than that. It allowed me to be able to prove to you that you are not being told the truth concerning this intriguing phenomena, which has become known as a Crop Circle or Pictogram. Not only the fact they are keeping the truth from you but the more insidious fact that they are going to a lot of trouble and expense to do so by inventing all sorts of crazy stories such as the Doug and Dave one in order to send you up the garden path as they say, knowing that this path will lead you away from the truth.

And why would they want to do that? Well perhaps we should draw the line and spend our time making our way through the next chapter discovering some of the reasons for this deliberate deceit.

9. ARE WE ALONE

In September 1994 I was on my fourth trip to the United States, and part of that time was spent in the lovely old town of Santa Fe in New Mexico. An excellent week of radio interviews, public meetings and workshops left a lot of very keen healers behind me when I went on to Albuquerque where, as I mentioned in Chapter 4 some time was spent on a TV interview at the New Mexico state fair. I also made a brief mention there of an interesting discussion I had with a government official at one of the stalls and promised I would record for you in a later chapter something of that discussion. This is the chapter I referred to, but I must ask you to bear with me for a short time while I describe to you something of what happened to bring that conversation about.

I have in front of me at the moment a copy of a newspaper. It is the Sunday Sante Fe New Mexican for September the 18th 1994. I kept this paper and bought it home with me for a very good reason. On the front page there is a headline which reads "CATTLE MUTILATIONS – Mystery on the Range". And it goes on to describe how since April 1993 one farmer has discovered 13 steers and 1 cow dead and mutilated – their sexual organs removed, their tongues cut out, and their anuses cored. Never is there a trace of blood, a tyre track or footprint even though the cattle are sometimes found far from the nearest road. There is quite a large area on the front page including two photographs concerning this strange happening, but at the bottom of the article are the words "please see research page 4".

If we turn over to page 4 we find that we have not only all of page 4 but also most of page 5 devoted to the same subject. What could be so important about this particular subject for 2 and a half pages of a newspaper to have been devoted to it. Obviously I can do no more than to give you a few short extracts from the article, but it is interesting to note that on the left side of page 4 there is a double column of short reports of animal mutilations in New Mexico spanning the period from August 28th 1975 – to August 30th 1994.

This long list begins with the following. August 28th: rancher Jimmy Wall discovers a dead calf, whose udder and sexual organs have been removed. August 31st: rancher Alver Simpson finds his prize bull mutilated, its sex organs cut out and its rectum cored. There are several other similar reports for that year but 1978 lists a total of eight similar discoveries in different areas, while 1979 came up with twenty four. If we add all of the reports of mutilated animals in this list which covers several states including Iowa, Missouri, Kansas and New Mexico to name a few, we find there is a total of fifty eight. But judging by the map they produced showing the areas in New Mexico that figure must represent a small portion of the total. The caption on that map reads "Since April 1993, ranchers have reported 46 cattle mutilations in northern New Mexico. Most of the cattle have been found west of Los Alamos near Valle Grande or the Eagle Nest area."

What is going on here and why? Perhaps your guess is as good as mine, but when I read a passage like most of the cattle have been found west of Los Alamos and in the Eagle Nest area, followed by a statement which tells us that snow that appeared blue in colour and caused some local residents to become burned or sick fell on Eagles Nest on May 17th 1955, I can't help but start wondering where the connection might lie. My mind goes back to 1985 when I was visiting Sante Fe. The man I was staying with on that occasion was a pilot and he took me up in a small plane to show me what the area looked like from the air. We covered quite a lot of country including one or two small towns and the Rio Grande. At one stage I asked him what the town was a short distance out to our right and what looked to be about 20 miles from Sante Fe. He told me that was Los Alamos, but he could not fly over there as that area was out of bounds for all aircraft. I already knew that Los Alamos was where the original atom bomb was developed for Hiroshima and Nagasaki, but this was 1985. What could be so secret that no planes were allowed to fly above the area. We did drive over there a few days later and drove past the long high security fences that surround the military area.

Was there some significance between what goes on in this area and the fact that so many mutilated animals were continually being discovered in that general vicinity. I am not suggesting that the military have anything to do with these strange happenings, but it would seem to me that the ones who are removing these organs from the animals are doing so with a view to taking them back to their own planet to test them in order to find what effect nuclear experiments etc being carried out in that area is having on animal life. In case you think I have suddenly lost my sanity when I wrote that last sentence I think perhaps I had better copy a little more from this extensive article. Needless to say all sorts of people, official and otherwise spent a lot of time investigating the phenomena, no one has come up with any positive answers to the mystery. But I think the following quote goes a long way toward backing up my own theories. "In 1947, the same year an unidentified flying object allegedly crashed near Roswell, William C de Baca found a mutilated cow on a ranch near La Cienega. According to his son, the cows sexual organs and udder were removed, it's anus cored out – typical of what would become known as the "*classic*" case of animal mutilation. At the time they thought it was coyotes. Coyotes kill cows, but I have never heard of a coyote sexually abusing the corpse, but it was not until 1967 the curious mystery gained widespread attention both in the US and across the world. That September, Lady, an Appaloosa Mare was found dead and horribly disfigured. The skin had been completely removed from the horses head and neck, the blood drained from her body and her major organs removed through what appeared to be surgical incisions. Strange lights doing what appeared to be impossible manoeuvres had been seen by local residents in the night sky before and after the horses death. That extraordinary twist sent the story across the Associated Press wires, and new phenomena was officially launched.

A laboratory scientist, Howard Burgess said he worked with officials from the University of Iowa's Veterinary Lab to determine what tool was used to excise the animals sexual organs and other body parts. A group of veterinary surgeons and lab technicians worked for more than eight hours on the carcass of a dead cow trying to duplicate incisions found on mutilated animals but could not. The head of the Vet Lab, one of the best in the US, said with a laugh "whoever was doing this, those fellows out there have more precision cutting tools than any one of our instruments here. We could not pinpoint an answer to who was doing it because they were doing something our best lab couldn't do".

You may be wondering why I appear to be labouring this whole business of mutilated animals, but believe me, there is a very good reason for this and we are heading in the right direction for me to be able to explain it for you. Apart from the actual healing work I do, I am really all about trying to get people to use what God gave them to think with. Most cannot be bothered about doing that. They figure it is much easier to simply accept what they are being told by Professor so and so or some other one of authority. They say to themselves he is the expert, he must know. But do not expect that to be the truth because that is about the last thing they want you to know.

If we now go back at long last to that conversation I had with the government official at the Mexico State Fair, then perhaps I can bring to you just one of the sort of situations I am referring to. This man was probably quite used to having discussions with the public and would be well aware that most of them would be quite willing to go along with whatever he told them and be accepted as being the truth because he was in a position to know. What he didn't realise when he asked me if there was anything I wanted to know about their work, was the fact that for once he was about to find himself up against someone who was not prepared to do that unless his explanation or information made good sense with what I was already aware of.

The particular stall I stopped at was staffed by two government paid men resplendent in the uniforms of what we would call in our country DOC or Department of Conservation. When I asked what sort of work they would actually do, he told me that their job was to assist farmers in any way they could. For instance, if a farmer was having a problem with dogs or wild coyotes killing their sheep or other animals, then they would be called on to the farmers property with a gun and eliminate the problem for them.

This mention of animals being attacked in some way immediately bought to my mind the two and a half page article I had read in the newspaper just two or three days ago. I said to him that I presumed he would know something about the mutilated animals that had been discovered over a long period of time on farms in his area. As I did so, I remember wondering to myself what sort of answer a government man would come up with. I did not think he would be likely to admit to me what I believed to be the truth, and I was certainly not disappointed in that respect. He assured me that he did know of these happenings, and when I pressed him for an explanation as to what he considered was taking place in these cases, I thought he looked a little concerned as if he was considering very carefully what answer he could give me to what I realised had been a difficult question for him to answer truthfully as a government employee.

After a few moments, he said rather quietly and slowly "Well I think its probably the coyotes that are doing it". Now I knew he was in trouble. I was aware that as a Government employee he needed to be very careful about what he had to say concerning such a thorny question as this one. My lady friend I was with was looking a little sideways at me by this time and I reckoned she was wondering whether I was about to be like the rest of the sheep and simply accept that answer and walk away. But knowing that answer made no sense whatsoever with the evidence I already had which proved that theory to be quite impossible, I was determined not to let him get away with telling me what he must have known to be nothing more than a deliberate lie.

The next few questions and answers went something like this

> "Do you really think the coyotes are doing this?",
> Again very slowly and thoughtfully "well yes I think so".
> "You obviously didn't read the article in the paper on Sunday?".
> "Yes I did actually".
> "You could not have read all of it then?"
> "Well yes I did"
> "And you still think the coyotes are still responsible for those incisions which the best vets in your country assured us they could not do, nor did they know of any instruments to remove organs in the way they had been removed. Surely this would mean the coyotes are far more cleaver than your veterinarians".

I felt there was rather an awkward moment for him as he glanced at my friend and back to me. I knew he was struggling with the dilemma he found himself in. Should he continue to stay with the explanation he had given me, an explanation I had obviously made to look very silly, or could he risk saying something he should not divulge as a Government employee, something like a thing called truth for instance. The last thing he would be supposed to give to the public. But he finally composed himself and made quite an amazing statement. He simply said even more slowly "Well, I must admit there has been a few strange lights around here at times."

At this stage, I almost felt sorry for him, but I knew I did not need to upset him any more by questioning any further. I had the answer I had been looking for. His last statement totally refuted his first one, so what more did I need. I could have asked him to explain what he meant, and to tell me where he felt the lights were coming from. But I reckoned I already knew the answer to that question anyway, and that he probably did to, but there was no way I was about to be cruel enough to push him into admitting any more of the truth which he had found so difficult to speak.

This little story I have just recorded for you is just one very small episode in the continuing saga of a bureaucracy which will go to any length in an effort to keep from the population, any thing which may upset or in any way be contrary to what you believe. And why would they do this you may well ask? There are many good reasons, most of which make their way back in one way or another to the mighty dollar. Just like the TV programme I wrote about in an earlier chapter. What loss is a few thousand dollars to a drug company if it becomes the means of sending many people who are attending some form of alternative clinic back to the doctor where he will then make out a prescription for some drug. They know that by using a well known comedian in such a programme in order to make all alternatives of healing look stupid, many viewers will believe what the "experts" say on that documentary and vow never to go near one of those practitioners of an art they have been able to show as being no more than a joke.

Every year in the US the taxpayer is bled to the tune of many billions of dollars so that the boys at NASA can have a wonderful time playing with their rockets. Do you really think they would want you to know that there are other methods by which man can travel the endless highways and byways of space by simply tapping into the ever present energy of the universe in the same way that people from other planets of other galaxies have obviously been doing for many centuries.

When the writer of Genesis spoke of the sons of God who came in unto the daughters of Earth and had intercourse with them, they must have been aware that these travellers would need to have a ship of some kind to travel in through the endless space. And just as Ezekiel gave his perfect description of what he saw in the sky as a wheel within a wheel, with eyes all about, so Job must have realised when he asked who these were who he saw flitting from cloud to cloud, they did not belong to this planet. But today, in spite of the literally thousands of people who have reported some wonderful sightings of these wheels within wheels flitting from cloud to cloud and even in some cases actually landing, the powers that be spend an incredible amount of tax payers money to convince those same tax payers that there has never been a genuine sighting of what has come to be called a UFO.

I find there are many people who have not made any real effort to study the Crop Circles who are quite convinced they are only found in England. While by far the greatest number have appeared in that country and have created more interest there than any where else, they have been discovered in many other countries throughout Europe, Unites States, and yes, even in New Zealand. For instance an extract from a report from the United States contains the following: "A Crop Circle appeared in an oat field at Herkimer, New York, on July 21, 1993. Another appeared at Kennewick, Washington in a wheat field on May 29th, 1993. Then on July the 3rd 1996, a beautiful Crop Circle appeared in a wheat field at Paulding". The writer went on to explain that he was a very good dowser and visited the Paulding site with his L wires. Apparently the circle was identical to the one I was on in Shrewsbury but instead of being 67 feet across, it was 93 feet. His description of it used the same words I would use to describe the Shrewsbury one. He said it was almost as if someone had used a giant cookie cutter to cut it out. The wheat stalks at the outer edge were standing tall and erect while right next to them the stalks were prone. And again, as I have already mentioned concerning Shrewsbury the stalks were laid down precisely in an anti clockwise direction.

He then goes on to mention the fact that he had always been a sceptic concerning UFO's but has now had to change his mind. He said that among the many people he talked to that evening while he was checking the circle with his rods, was a young woman who described the experience she had the evening the crop circle appeared. She was driving to work when an object flew past above her. It was so bright she could not look directly at it. As it passed her, the car lights went out and the engine stopped. After it moved away a short distance ahead of her the lights came on and the engine started up again. Several miles down the road she pulled in to a restaurant and found the lights there had also been extinguished for a few seconds.

Perhaps I may have some readers who may have never heard of anything like this happening, but this can only mean that you have never bothered to make any effort to investigate the overwhelming evidence concerning such phenomena. There have been many similar reports of car engines stopping and lights being temporarily extinguished from several countries. There never appears to be any structural damage to any electrical equipment as they always return to normal as soon as the light, or should I dare to stay, the UFO moves a short distance away. It would appear that the ship has a strong field around it just as an ordinary magnet as we know also has. We know that if we move a magnet past a length of wire an electrical current is set up in that wire, and of course this is basically how we generate all our electricity so it should not be to difficult to imagine a ship with a very strong field of some kind, and not necessarily a magnetic field as we know it, but possibly some kind of field we are not yet even aware of or capable of producing. As the ship passes something like a car which relies on electrical current for both the running of it's engine and it's lights, the car would come within the orbit of that field and create perhaps a resistance to the normal flow of the energy through the cars electrical system, and of course we know what would happen. And apparently it does.

Sounds like science fiction or maybe a miracle or magic. Well, all I can say about that is Arthur C Clarke got it right in one short sentence. And if you don't mind Arthur I would like to quote that masterpiece here for the benefit of my readers "Any sufficiently advanced technology is indistinguishable from magic".

And I find that a magic statement. I realise my younger readers may not see it quite in the way that I do. But you see, with just a few months to go before I will be celebrating the big 80 I have seen many changes take place on the planet. As I watch a colour TV today, or look at what my sons and grandsons and grand-daughters have stored on a little disc and can bring up on the screen of their computers at the touch of a button I am not sure whether I should refer to these things and many more which we take for granted today, as miracles or magic. But I can assure you that when I was a boy 75 years or so ago, those two words would barely have been strong enough to use to describe them. It is more likely that many, particularly the older people of that time would have been reaching for something more like "witchcraft" or works of the devil. Such is the progress which has been made in that respect in my life time, and I have no doubt that providing we do not make the fatal mistake of becoming so clever, that we limit ourselves as a species, then you young ones will see even greater advancements by the time you reach my age.

But be aware, I was not joking when I wrote that last sentence. As a boy I could have never imagined for one moment that owing to a thing called "science", (and I make no excuses for putting that in parenthesis) we would ever become so clever that we would be able to wipe from the face of the earth several thousand innocent people, also with the touch of a button, but I presume that was about all that was needed when Enola Gay arrived over Hiroshima. Of course, that was merely an experiment compared to what we could do today if the "need" should arise. And may God help us if it ever does, for then science will really be able to show us what they can do. I always feel that the most important letter in that word, science, is the N. You may well ask me why I would think that. Simply because every time I look at it I see that letter representing the word "negative". A low frequency negative science which can only leave in its wake many levels of pollution, destruction and death.

If we wish to avoid this then we must look toward the true science, the science of the higher frequency energy, and the constructive, instead of the destructive. In case you are finding it difficult to understand what I am trying to say here let me give you just one suggestion of the sort of thing I am referring to. Of all the organs I have worked on over the years, the liver would be by far the most common. Many times I found that people who have come into my healing room looking very tired have blood which is full of poison and a liver which is in a very bad state. Time and again I have found on questioning them, they work perhaps in an orchard, a kiwifruit one in particular, where a great deal of poison is sprayed every so often to kill any insects which may harm the fruit.

As soon as my hand enters the energy field around the leg and I think to myself that I will clear the blood and the artery beneath it, I find that it is almost impossible to move my hand at all, such is the resistance which is created by the negativity within that field. And how did it get there? As a result of that negative science with its mistaken belief that the way for us to exist is to poison everything that gets in our way. And how do we overcome or remove the damage to the human body which that policy has created? Oh yes, I know how the same science attempts to do it. You will go to the doctor with your problems and he will prescribe some drug or some chemical in order to attempt to fight the result of the chemical that has caused the problem in the first place. What a vicious circle we follow. Especially when as all to often happens, the chemical he gives you creates a side effect so the doctor has to write you out a prescription to fight the one the first one created. But that is not the answer. You cannot fight one negative thing within another. The answer is to use something positive to remove the negativity. And so we turn to the opposite vibration. The positive, healing, natural, universal energy, the true science to reverse the situation which their negative science has spawned.

It is my belief that there are many living beings cruising the highways of the universe who have already long since come to this realisation, and have thrown away the idea that to leave a planet you must create a force powerful enough for you to force your way, I was about to say, upwards, but that in itself would have been a negative. So let me change that to a more appropriate word, outward. For there is no "UP" only out. And when we can finally get around to the understanding that there is nothing but energy throughout an endless universe, energy in it's many forms and frequencies of vibration, then we too, we members of the kindergarten race we call man, will be able to lift ourselves above this level of dog eat dog existence which our present level of science appears to thrive on. Then like those who have been cruising the universe for so long in their "wheel within a wheel" we will know that it is not necessary to fight this thing we call gravity, and in doing so, pollute the atmosphere of our planet in the inexcusable way in which we are presently doing.

We speak of miracles, but what is a miracle. For me that which we call a miracle is no more than a perfectly normal happening which takes place within the frame work of a particular universal law which we do not yet understand simply because we do not yet have any knowledge of that law. But as we climb the ladder of evolvement and move from the kindergarten to a higher grade so we will learn to know these higher laws and to be aware that by making use of them, then we will be able to perform what we would previously have considered to be miracles. We will know that contrary to believing that it is necessary to force ourselves against what we tend to think of the enemy, the force of gravity, with the understanding of energy we will find it to be our ally as we learn to meld with it and use it in a positive way to assist us in our endeavours to move out in to those same highways and byways of space which others have enjoyed cruising through for so long.

A resident of Wiltshire in England, where the largest number of Crop Circles have been recorded over several years had this to say "Some of the Crop Circles are a hoax but some of them are genuine and maybe they are made by aliens. How else can you account for them? Three years ago, a Crop Circle appeared in the meadow behind our house. It was not there when we went to bed but it was there in the morning. And every clock in the house had stopped. Not just the electric ones and the oven timer, but the wind-up ones as well. Plus both of our wrist watchers. How do you account for that?"

He explains that he can't account for it, but he has to admit that curious things do happen in that part of Britain. I must admit that like him I can't account for it either but I do know for sure that it was not done by Doug and Dave. But the point is these things are happening, and surely our scientists instead of continuing to ignore them because they know that such things are impossible, would do better to put some of their time and energy into trying to discover the universal laws which make it possible for such things to take place. While I don't find the stopping of the electric clocks any great problem to understand as this is little different to cutting the current in a car engine and extinguishing its lights, when we look at the stopping of wind-up ones with no electrical circuits to be blocked then this is surely something we need to give even more consideration to. It means that someone out there knows enough about energy to be able to use it in some way to even cancel out at least temporarily the ability of a wind-up spring with all its stored energy waiting to be released from being able to do so.

And of course, a study of crop circles brings the realisation that they also know how to use energy in some seemingly miraculous way to bend thousands of stalks of corn, wheat or rape. And I added that last one for a very good reason. Not just because some of them are created in fields of rape, but because rape has a rather different property to the others. While it may be quite difficult to bend, wheat or corn stalks at 90 degrees a short distance above the ground and lay them flat on the ground without them breaking and still having the ability to continue growing as I saw thousands doing in the circles I visited in 1996, it is totally impossible to do so with rape. Rape is very much like celery and every cook knows you cannot bend a stalk of celery 90 degrees without having it crack and break. And rape is no better in that respect. Because of it's brittleness it is quite impossible to do that with it, but apparently someone out there has not heard of that word impossible, because they are sending down a beam of energy and bending the stalk at 90 degrees as if no one has ever told them they cannot do that.

I never cease to be amazed at the number of times I hear some scientist or astronomer talking about how they are listening with thousands of dollars worth of equipment, just in case there may happen to be someone else out there somewhere. Where have they been these last few years? Have they been hiding themselves away in a tunnel somewhere in total darkness to ensure that they do not see something which they cannot understand and would therefore look a little silly if they had to admit what they saw was something they could not explain. Is it too much to ask them to put aside for a little while their inflated egos and admit that there is much which they do not yet understand. Of course, it would be infinitely more difficult for them to agree that there were others who frequently come into the atmosphere who obviously do understand the laws by which these things can be made to take place.

And surely we have something here that is totally akin to the situation we have concerning the sort of healing work which healers such as myself are doing. Medical science KNOWS that it is impossible to simply move your hands over a body more often than not, without even touching the body and not only discovering where a group of cells in that body has become out of phase therefore making that body ill, but also apply energy with those hands which will actually restore that group of cells to their normal condition so that the body will now be at ease instead of diseased.

Lets try putting these two apparently very different phenomena together and see if we can find some sort of parallel between them. I am aware that it does seem a long way between bending thousands of stalks of some crop without even touching them, and restoring cells in an ailing body. But if we just think about this a little we will realise that they do have more in common than perhaps we first thought. For a start they both fit into the same category in respect to the way they are looked upon by orthodox science. In this respect they are both considered to be quite impossible and therefore not worth wasting any time or effort on to investigate. Of course there is a very good reason for this. Neither or them fits into the very low frequency level of vibration which our science is limited to.

How then can they expect to begin to understand the science of the higher frequency energies when they will not accept that any such thing even exists, leave alone the fact that more and more people are not only becoming aware of it, but because of their belief in it are actually using it in a positive way to help an ever increasing number of suffering humanity to return their bodies to normal health. A few months ago I was watching a programme on TV which concerned a Russian doctor living in the United States but was not allowed to practice there. He claimed that when he looked at a patient he could actually see inside the body and pick up visually where most problems were. Extensive experiments were carried out in attempt to disprove this claim. A patient was diagnosed in the normal way and was also checked out by a chiropractor for any structural problems. The patient was then taken into a room at the other end of the building, while the Russian doctor who he had never met remained in the room with the other medical people and two cameras.

He was then given the name of the patient, and he sat down and "viewed" the body in the other room. It was not long before he began to describe what he was seeing in that body and it became very obvious by the look on the faces of the medical people that he was scoring some very direct hits. As he spoke you could see them referring to the notes they had made when they examined the body physically, and it was easy to see that every now and then they were quite shocked by what they were hearing as they pointed to something they had written earlier and shook their heads as if they were not believing what they were hearing. For instance he said he could see a scar on the heart where the patient had suffered some sort of attack and the doctors had to admit that he had a heart attack a few years ago which had left a scar there.

I realise this may sound quite amazing to some people, but for me who has had many wonderful personal experiences working with several people, who possessed similar abilities, the only amazing thing about it is the fact that because all these wonderful gifts have been scoffed at for so long and considered by those who still insist on remaining within the boundaries of their "so called" science, the general public knows nothing of them. What wasted opportunities exist on our planet. There are many out there who have similar gifts but are considered to be just a little strange. When I try to explain to a doctor that if a body is laying on the couch in front of me, I run my hands through the energy field and find out exactly where the problem is, they think I am crazy. But if I was to suggest I do not even need the patient there in that form but can merely visualise her laying there by thinking about her name, and continue to do the same work of finding the problem and removing it even if the body is on the other side of the world, then most would be quite sure that I am either crazy or just a charlatan.

The fact that it has happened many times and at least two of the recipients have been so pleased with the result that they have sent me Airline Tickets to fly to their homes on the other side of the world does not appear to have any effect on them. They know it is impossible so do not want to hear about it. Of course they are right, such things are impossible as long as you are still down there on that low frequency level of understanding which orthodox science relies on. A very limited low frequency vibration. If only they had listened to Nicola Tesla, the great inventor, who was so many years ahead of his time when he discovered alternating current, and many other wonderful inventions. "In that single decade when science first begins to investigate the non-physical, they will make more progress in that decade than they have made in the past century".

Whether it be using energy to restore the damaged cells of a human being or an animal, whether you are using energy to propel a ship through the endless highways of space, or using it to create a beautiful Crop Circle in a wheat field with the intention of making people start thinking for themselves, it is still high frequency energy you are using. That non-physical which Tesla spoke about. There is nothing else but energy, and it is free. Whether it be the energy locked up in a single atom or the energy which whirls a galaxy of a thousand million stars through endless space, it is still energy. Boundless and free. Able to be used in a negative way to destroy, or equally capable of being used in a positive way to create. When will we step away from the former and recognise the latter. Splitting the atom, the very building blocks of nature must be the ultimate in the degradation to which our scientists have sunk. The 175,000 innocent victims of Hiroshima and Nagasaki would certainly agree with that I am sure, if they were alive to tell you. Destruction, construction, to destroy to create, negative or positive, low frequency physical level, high frequency non-physical. The choice is ours. But how long can we afford to wait for this change? We need it now before our continual poisoning of Planet Earth and her environs by a science which refuses to look outside their boundaries brings about an irreversible condition which will make it impossible for Earthmother to sustain her children.

And judging by the video I have just been watching this morning it would seem that there is still plenty going on in secret behind closed doors which makes one wonder why they are afraid to tell the taxpayer, who of course is paying for it all, just what it is all about. They mentioned how President Clinton had declared a huge exclusion zone around Area 51 in the Nevada Desert where the stealth fighter was developed. A man by the name of Robert claims that he worked there at one time and said the security was quite bizarre. Everywhere he went he was followed by security guards. Sometime after he left his job he caused a sensation by revealing he had been ordered to investigate the propulsion system of a captured alien spacecraft. He described the shape of the craft as being like two inverted dishes (something like a wheel within a wheel?). Authorities immediately denied his claim and have tried to erase his identity. An investigative reporter took on the case, but they still denied any knowledge of ever having him there. Then they showed us the phone book for the lab, and there was his name listed in it. Four different polygraph tests showed that in each case he was telling the truth and could not be tripped up in any way. This included his statements concerning his having worked at the base, about seeing the flying saucers, and working on anti-gravity propulsion systems.

I like that last bit. You see I have always believed that for every action there is a reaction, for every force in nature there is an equal and opposite force, and I feel sure that if science would change their attitude toward this sort of understanding and put more time into discovering more about energy instead of trying to build bigger and better air polluting rockets, then we would find we could go with nature instead of forcing ourselves against her in our ignorance of her benevolence when she is treated with respect. Our friend Robert on that tape finished up by telling us that both he and his wife had been threatened on more than one occasion. Apparently they had not liked him saying his job had been what is called back engineering. Not making or inventing something, but trying to find out how something worked, as the technology they were dealing with did not yet exist within the framework of our present science.

Take a look at the picture on Page **123** . This Crop Circle appeared at Milk Hill in Wiltshire on 8th August 1997, in a field of wheat. It measured 246 feet by 216 feet. I took a rough count of the small circles along the inner and outer edges and came up with a figure around two hundred. Our friends Doug and Dave with their board attached to a steel handle must have been extremely busy that night. They must be wonderful mathematicians and engineers to work out such an incredible shape in the dark of night, and they must be great athletes to be able to jump from one circle to the place where they want to make the next as it is easy to see there are no tracks between them which would show up if they had walked from one to the next. I happen to know this to be true because a careful study has been done in England to prove this point, and found that no matter how carefully someone walked through a field of wheat, they could not do so without their path showing up very clearly in any aerial photo taken such as this one. Perhaps the most difficult thing for me to understand about all this is how supposedly intelligent people can deliberately ignore this sort of evidence and still say that there is no way these Pictograms could have been created by ET's simply sending down energy from a ship above the area and must have been done by somebody such as Doug and Dave. How little they know about energy and the miracles which we could perform if only we would open our closed minds to the endless possibilities which await our discovery.

10. SPREADING THE LIGHT

Having just written the heading to this new chapter, I find myself looking at it and wondering whether I may have made a mistake in calling it by that name. I must admit it does sound a little bit like I am about to become all religious and start preaching to you like some great revivalist. Let me assure you that will not be the case. Some of my writings contain a degree of the sort of fervour with which those people bring their beliefs to all those who will listen, but I would hope my reasons for doing so would not be quite the same as theirs. From what I have seen of them it would seem to me that the great majority of these people are doing this simply because some other carried away evangelist has infiltrated their mind with a particular religious belief to the extent where they now find it impossible to use to any great extent what God gave them to think with.

They cease to be a thinking individual and merely continue to perpetuate the thought pattern which has been implanted in their minds by another. And of course this can apply equally to many different religious beliefs, whether it be Muslim, Christian or one of the hundreds of different sects who have convinced themselves that theirs is the only true religion and therefore the only path to God. Of course, when people realise that, as I think I have already mentioned, the kingdom of God is within you, and as Jesus told the people "ye are Gods" then obviously they will become aware that they do not need any one of those religions to show them the pathway to God, because they will be fully aware that they are already there. With the recognition of your Godliness comes the realisation that you are already one with Him and can cease the endless searching for the inner peace we so desire. "I am in Him, and he is in me". Why do we in our ignorance continue to doubt for one moment that Jesus really meant every statement he made. Surely they were made for your enlightenment, "Why doubtest thou, O ye of little faith?"

My word, I am beginning to sound like an evangelist after all. And it's strange, because that is not the line of thought I actually began this chapter with when I wrote up that heading. It was more along the lines of writing about what I have been doing over the past years and why I have been doing it, and continuing to do so in this my eightieth year. But I make no excuses for having written those few paragraphs. When something like this rolls off the end of my pen, then I am aware that someone knows there will be some reader or readers who will realise those words were just the ones they needed in order to trigger within them the recognition of their true soulself within, and by doing so, start them off on a whole new well lit path where truth becomes reality, and the old beliefs will fall away. Belief can be a stumbling block which can trip you up in the shadows of uncertainty, but a recognition of truth will set your feet firmly on a lighted path where doubt no longer holds sway over your life.

It was my intention at this stage to begin recording for you some of my recollections of last years trip to the US, but just as I was about to do so, I noticed a large envelope at the end of my desk and decided to have a check to see what it contained. Long before I start writing a book I clip interesting items from newspapers or magazines and put them in envelopes in case they should come in handy as reference material when I do get around to writing the next one. When I picked up this particular envelope, I noticed I had written one word on it. It simply said Religion. Judging by what I have written so far in this chapter I immediately felt it was not by accident that my eye just happened to notice that envelope at this time. On opening it up, and looking at its contents, it became quite clear that there was a good reason for doing so, and I knew that U.S. would have to wait a little longer while I gleaned a few interesting extracts from the cuttings within it.

The first one I picked up had a caption which read, "Vatican admits 2,000 years of sin". Could I be reading correctly? Did this really mean that one of the world's greatest religions was about to admit that for the past 2,000 years their faithful followers had actually been sinners. Surely this could not be. But let me quote a few lines from it, then I will simply let you be the judge of that.

"The Pope and the world's Cardinals began a secret two day meeting last night to discuss the Catholic Church's future. They plan to mark the year 2,000 by admitting past failings such as the Inquisition.

The Cardinals are discussing a 25 page confidential memorandum sent to them by Vatican Secretary of State, Cardinal Angelo Sodamo, and reflecting some of the Popes ideas for the celebrations. The memo was obtained from Vatican sources. One Section says the year 2,000 could be a particularly propitious and privileged chance for the Church to recognise "the dark side of its history" and the failings of some of its members in the first 2,000 years of its life.

How can one remain silent about the many forms of violence perpetrated in the name of faith? – wars of religion, tribunals of the Inquisition and other forms of violations of the rights of persons.

During the Inquisition, which reached its height in the 16th century to counter the Protestant Reformation, Christians who were considered heretics were tortured and killed if they did not recant. Many were burned at the stake. The memo specifically cites the case of Italian astronomer Galileo, who was condemned by the Inquisition in the 17th Century for asserting the Earth revolved around the Sun. They condemned his theories because they ran contrary to the Bibles declaration, "God fixes the Earth upon its foundation not to be moved forever".

There is more to this article, but I feel I have already given you more than enough to convince you there was a good reason for writing the sentence just back a little which begins with the words, "belief can be a stumbling block" etc. Surely this is the perfect example of a large number of people having their minds so controlled that it did not even occur to them that their belief was exactly that, their belief. As we are well aware today and poor old Galileo was already aware back in the seventeenth century, their belief had nothing in common whatsoever with truth, but such was the fear engendered within them by an all powerful religious fraternity which had told them, "Thou shalt believe this or else" that they were prepared to be a part of the torturing, the imprisoning, the burning at the stake of anyone who dared to question those beliefs.

You may like to step back a little to where you will see near the beginning of this chapter the sentence which begins "they cease to be a thinking individual" and I am sure that if you did not realise why I was writing that when you read it the first time, you will do so now.

Perhaps some of my readers are saying to themselves, "Yes but that was hundreds of years ago, we are more civilised than that now". Are you quite sure about that. I hate to keep asking you to go back and read again some of what has been written here, but either before you read the next quotation I am about to copy for you, or after you have read it if you wish, I suggest you check on the sentence which explains what the Inquisition was all about, finishing with the words "many were burned at the stake".

The second news cuttings I picked up in that envelope had nothing to do with Catholic versus Protestant argument of a few hundred years ago or the right for the individual to have his or her own choice of thought pattern at that time, but was right up to date in the late 1990's. "Sectarian arsonists killed three Catholic children in an attack on a house in the town of Ballymoney early yesterday. Chief Inspector Terry Shevlin called it a sickening and brutal murder. ("suffer the little children to come unto me"). Protestant extremists have launched a wave of violence in retaliation for the banning of a street parade which members of the Orange Order wanted to hold a week ago through a Catholic enclave in the town of Portadown. Ballymoney was one of several towns hit by sectarian violence this week."

Now what was that you were saying about being more civilised, enlightened, free thinking, or whatever it was you are believing we are today? And please do not get the idea that Catholic ard Protestant religions are the only ones which still insist on controlling the thinking pattern of the masses in order to hold sway over them and control them like a sheep farmers well trained dogs would have total control over his flock.

Can you believe the headline I saw at the top of the next little piece of paper I drew out of my envelope? "Paper bags threat to Islam, say Taleban". Paper bags: I am sure that like me you are asking yourself how paper bags could possibly be a threat to any religion, no matter how 'way out' they might be. But here is their incredible explanation.

"Paper bags have been banned by Afghanistan Muslim fundamentalists in their campaign to impose pure Islamic law. (Translation: In their campaign to poison and take control of the minds of the masses (Author)). We respect paper whether it is written on or not. We have announced that people should not use paper bags or put paper on the rubbish tip, said the information Minister of the Taleban administration. The Taleban said there might be words from the Holy Koran on the paper, which might then be thrown away, and that would be an insult to the Koran.

Since the edict there has been a rush to buy toilet paper by people unsure how wide the ban would go. The fundamentalists took power in September and have since barred women from the workplace and decreed that Government workers grow beards".

Surely I hardly need to make any comment on a statement such as this. I accept that my reader will have enough intelligence of his or her own to be filled with his or her own disgust at such pronouncements without me having to add mine. That is of course, unless you happen to be unfortunate enough to have been caught in the trap that has been set for you, and have joined the flock of sheep known as Muslim fundamentalists. In which case you may be in favour of the strict orders the Taleban militia have decreed for their second class citizens, the ones who happen to have arrived on the Planet in this incarnation in a physical body marked 'female'.

"Afghanistan's Islamic Taleban Militia has ordered Kabul residents to screen windows in their homes to ensure that women cannot be seen from the street. Householders have until April 9th to comply with the rules or face undisclosed punishment according to Sharia Islamic law. A Taleban official in the Attorney Generals office in Kabul said that women's faces could corrupt men. The face of a woman is a source of corruption for men who are not related to them, said the official explaining that women should be veiled in public places."

I am appalled to find that the male leaders of a religion can admit to being so weak minded and apparently totally unable to have any control over their emotions, that they must pass laws which will make the opposite sex hardly more than outcasts. They also mention that women will be banned from most workplaces and most education will be halted for girls and women. I said outcasts, but in the light of that last statement, it would seem I should add to that, the word slaves. I would suggest to these men, or should I use the more correct word, bigots, that if they have a problem with women, then the one sure way of finding the problem, and the means to remove it if they so desire, is not to look at the women, for they are not the real problem, but to take a good long hard look in the mirror, for there they will see, looking back at them the source of all their problems. And if they have the courage and the intelligence to look deeply enough into the reflection they see before them then they will know that within that same image which is the creator of their problems, lies all the answers they could ever need to solve them.

Create and destroy. Destroy and create. Are these not the opposing sides of everything that ever takes place within the realms of creation. From the tiniest of microbal life to the creating and destroying and recreating again and again, the stars, the supernova that explodes after a billion years of life, only to reform and build again from the dust of its demise.

So within the mind of man even the greatest of bigots, lies that seed of creation that can be nurtured and developed to grow into a thing of beauty. Look within, for here lies all the answers we could ever need to solve every problem we have ever been faced with, including the ones we have spawned due to our ignorance of our true soulself within and our ability to use for the benefit of mankind the incredible intellect which cries out for us to recognise.

Even in our own little country we have those who would desire to control the minds of their fellow beings and tell them what they should believe and what they should not believe. A newspaper article just last year reported on a group who work under the name of Cultwatch. While I agree that I would be in favour of helping those who have joined up with, or are considering joining a cult such as the Heavens Gate in San Diego where 39 members took their own lives in 1997, obviously devoid of any control of their own minds after the brainwashing they were suffering from, one look at the beliefs of this group who call themselves "Cultbusters" would surely brand them as being equally as dangerous as any of the very cults they have set out to bust.

"Auckland's own cult-busters are based in a simple white house on the edge of the City's Bible belt at Mt Roskill. Trevor Mander, Operations Manager of Cultwatch works from a small room stacked with books, pamphlets and a computer. A stereo plays Christian music in the background. Mr Mander sees the work as vitally important. Cultwatch is a Christian based organisation that draws its workers from across the ecumenical divides.

New Zealand has about 200 Cults, including the many New Age movements that have sprung up during the 1990's. There are many splinter groups going well all over the place. New Zealand is quite an involved base for New Age Cults. He puts groups which believe in reincarnation, crystal power, holistic health, and inner healing under New Age".

There is much more, but surely I have already quoted enough to prove my point when I say that such a group as this is equally as dangerous as any of the cults they have set out to bust. Perhaps we need a group of cult busters to bust cults such as this. Reincarnation, crystal power, holistic health and inner healing. Can you believe what you are reading here? It would seem that bigots come in all shapes and forms, and even in our own locality. If these are Christians, then I can only ask may God protect me from Christians. The many people I have shown how to use the loveforce to help their fellowman in need and have now formed into a group we call "Healers Unlimited" must surely be in the forefront of those who this cult of Cultbusters would consider to be a threat to humanity. What sort of twisted minds could consider for one moment that one who gives his or her all over many years, as I have done, to reach out their hands and ask for this healing to flow to an ailing body to bring new health, hope and upliftment of body, mind and soul could in any way be a threat to anyone.

Perhaps I should rephrase that, because the truth is we are a threat to quite a few people on this planet. As so many of those we work with to bring that new health to are often those who have failed to be given much assistance after spending a lot of time and money working with orthodox medical practice, it is true that if we then find the source of the problem and remove it, that patient is no longer making return visits to their doctor. So yes, in that respect, you could say, we are a threat to the medical profession. Dollars do not flow in from patients who no longer have the need to visit them, but worse than that, those doctors who are not being visited by their ex patients are not writing out prescriptions for the Multi Million Dollar drug companies. They are the ones who we threaten most of all, and I am sure they are the ones who would like to bust us.

Why else would you put a comedian on a serious documentary about alternative methods of healing which do not use drugs if it was not an attempt to bust those practitioners who were not prescribing them? But the Cultbusters we have just been reading about have not formed their group because we threaten their pocket. They are demanding that you must believe that their 'truth' is the only one. You must not dare to think for yourselves and consider for one moment that what they, with their "Christian" beliefs, tell you is the whole truth and nothing but the truth could be in any way controversial.

We appear to have travelled around a lot since I first set up that title at the beginning of this chapter, but as I mentioned earlier, there is always a good reason for what I find written on the paper in front of me, so while there may be some readers who do not feel they have gained by reading it, I am quite confident that there will be plenty of others who will be saying something like "Good on him, it's about time someone woke the people up to what goes on around us".

While I have already recorded for you some of the exciting times I was privileged to experience in Vermont this time last year (while working with a doctor), there are still other things which occurred on that trip which are well worthy of a mention here. My first stop was LA where I stayed for a few days with the same Tim and Suzanne I had visited in '94. During those few days we held a public meeting with a workshop on each of the two following days. Here too I had the pleasure of having an old friend of Suzanne's who was a doctor come and join with us and discover that he, too, was also capable of reaching out his hands to a patient and feeling the flow of the energy through them, which allowed him, like his ancient predecessor Hippocrates, to pull and draw away aches and diverse impurities.

On the last evening we had three couches lined up in their large lounge while 23 of the keenest students from the previous classes took their turn at giving healing to anyone who needed it. I always find it to be extremely rewarding when I can stand back at a time such as this and watch people who have lived all of their life without having ever imagined for one moment, that they had, laying dormant within them, the ability to be used as channels for healing energy, now demonstrating that they have crossed the great divide from ignorance, and are bringing new levels of health to those in need. In all my years of healing many thousands of people, I used to think that nothing could be more rewarding than seeing the response of my patients to the healing I had given them, but to know that I have been able to pass this ability on to several others brings rewards and joy of an infinitely greater level. I know that for each one who discovers their true potential, there will be many others who, in the months or years to come will gain much from this ones newly found gift of healing.

From Los Angeles across the US and north to Vermont was a long trip but the one hour spent at a radio station, a few minutes of interview on TV3 on the early morning news in Burlington, the large public meeting, the several workshops and the healers I left behind me, plus those I worked with in Florence, Massachusetts were rewards beyond belief. I have already in an earlier chapter told you something about working with Dr Anderson, but there were many other highlights to my visit to Vermont and one or two of them would certainly not go amiss here.

On one occasion I worked on a dog belonging to two friends who had made the long drive from New York to visit me. The dog was muzzled just in case it should decide to bite me when it felt the energy. While some have actually made a little snap at my hand when I have whipped something away from them, I do not think any of them were really trying to bite me, but were just saying in the only way they know how, "I felt that". This particular dog had a problem with his head, and as my hand approached that area and entered the negative energy it became very obvious that he was feeling something happening which felt strange to him. Then my guide Dr Wilbur Sargesson stepped in and took over as he sometimes does if he feels it is necessary to bring in an even higher frequency energy to clear a particularly serious problem. When this happens my hands fly like the wings of a humming bird, moving so fast that sometimes it is almost impossible to see them at all. See photo front of cover, this was one of those occasions, and the dog's reaction to this was quite amazing. When I started to work on him, he began shivering as if in fear, but almost immediately he calmed right down and looked as if he was quite enjoying what was happening to him.

I had almost forgotten about this particular event until just a few days ago when a similar thing occurred. But this time it was not a dog I was working on, but a small boy between two and three years old. His mother had brought him into my healing room with her, and while I gave her some healing the boy sat quietly looking at some small childrens books which I keep there for just such an occasion. Everything went fine, until it was his turn to lay on the couch for some healing. The mother struggled to get him to lie down as he yelled and screamed the "I don't want to" story I have already heard a number of times before from very unwilling patients. However the mother felt that it was very necessary for me to do what I could for a particular problem he was suffering from, so while she held the torso down I held one leg and worked along with the hand to clear the blood as best I could. I was just wondering how I was going to manage to work my way through the whole body in this way, when as happened with the dog in Vermont almost one year ago to the day my doctor guide stepped in. My hands began to fly like a whirlwind, and what the boy saw I do not know, but what I do know is that his mother was absolutely amazed as she suddenly found she was able to lift her hands from her son and stand back and look at the little angel we now saw laying in front of us.

Just what had happened to bring about this incredible instant change from a screaming, probably very frightened little boy to a motionless body which looked up at me and never took his eyes off me for one moment while I worked through the whole of the torso in order to remove his problem we may never know, but I think it would be a pretty safe bet to suggest he was suddenly confronted with an image of my Doctor Sargesson. In some way this sudden change of scene for him appeared to remove all fear of what was taking place and he became perfectly happy to lay there and gaze at whatever it was he was seeing for as long as I needed to clear whatever I came up against in his aura. When I had done this I asked him if he would like to turn over on his tummy, so that I could check his back. This he did immediately without one word passing his lips, while his mother just shook her head in disbelief at what she was seeing.

Many times over the years I have had many very good reasons for giving a lot of thought to just how much young children actually see without ever saying anything to their parents or whatever adults may be there at the time. The little Maori girl who saw me throw away the "lump of black meat" as I drew the cancer away from her mothers tummy made no mention at all of what she had seen at the time, yet about an hour later she had just casually mentioned to her parents that she had not seen other doctors do that. What had been going on in her mind during that time? I do not think for one moment that she had even considered that her parents had not seen what she had been looking at. Nobody had told her she was not supposed to 'imagine' that she saw such things because they did not exist. But the tragedy is that as she grows up and she goes to school with all the other sheep in the pen she will soon learn that it does not pay to be different. She will soon realise that others are looking at her and treating her as if she is a little strange. Other children can be quite nasty towards someone they consider to be different to themselves and it is not long before they realise the only way to avoid such treatment is to conform and become one of them.

But if we can go out and spread the light of understanding a little wider and help people to understand that truth in all its simplicity is the only thing which is of any consequence in our quest for peace and harmony for Planet Earth and her struggling humanity, then we will have lifted our brothers and sisters just another rung or two up that long ladder of evolvement which each and every living soul on the planet has come here to climb. Perhaps the most distressing part of this is the fact that so many are in no way aware that there is a ladder to climb. All too many are stuck with the erroneous belief that they are a physical being here today and gone tomorrow, back to the dust from which they came. Their understanding of their true soulself within can be as little as nil, and so they falsely believe that they may as well have a good time while they are here, and too bad if someone gets in their way. If only they could know that first and foremost they are Spirit, a living soul, a spark of God, temporarily residing in a physical form in a physical world for a few short years in order to learn lessons which will raise the vibration of that soul to a higher level where they can become one with what we so vaguely refer to as God.

If you are one who has already made the effort to gain this understanding where your body vibrates with the joy of the recognition of truth, then I implore you to not hide your light under a bushel as they say in the Bible, but let all who would wish to come in to its presence be welcomed and invited to share this joy with you. I have just arrived back this afternoon from a city called Wanganui. Friday morning some time was spent on one of their local radio stations, and in the evening we held a public meeting in a hall where I showed 50 colour slides covering many aspects of the use of energy. This was followed by a demonstration of Magnetic Healing on a patient, while Saturday was spent running a workshop in the morning where I was able to show about twenty people how to become healers. The evening saw me standing in front of another group and going through the same procedure once again. Many of those have assured me they will be getting together in groups to continue to practice what I have shown them, and I have no doubt that in the months and years to come many people will find new health at the hands of those students as they use their newfound ability to be used as channels for that ever present universal energy which cries out for you to recognise it and to use it for the general good of mankind. Let your light shine for all to see.

Checking my notes for August 19th '98, I find a very interesting story which I feel is well worth telling. Copying from these notes, for that day, I find they read like this: - "9:30 to 12:30 am – 21 people. Another great group containing 'Healers Unlimited'". From this comment it is obvious that once again I had found that almost all of those 21 students had discovered that they too, can be used as channels for the healing energy. This is the really rewarding part of my work. To watch them come up to the patient on the couch, and to see so many of them suddenly finding that they are having difficulty bringing their hands together due to the build up of pressure between them.

But while that short note from my diary does bring back some very fond memories of the proceedings on that day, the rest of my notes bring with them a degree of satisfaction for me which is difficult to put into words. They concern a lady who had been to one of my classes the previous day and had rung my host Lisa to tell her what had happened when she arrived home from the meeting. Her cat was suffering from Feline Aids, so she thought that as I had told the students this healing worked very well on animals, she may as well try her newfound ability on the cat. She put it up on the table and placed her hands around it, gradually bringing them together close to the cat's body. She said she could feel the pressure building up between her hands until it became difficult to bring them together just as it had been when she was working on the patient at the meeting just an hour or two earlier. Finally she managed to do this and as she lifted this very strong negative energy away from the cat it was as if she actually had something quite heavy in her hands. She turned toward her left and vigorously threw whatever she was holding into that corner of the room.

She was amazed to see the cat jump off the table, and with front paws thrashing at whatever it was she had thrown away, chased it right into the corner. Once again we are reminded of our 6 year old Maori girl talking about the lump of black meat she had seen me throw into the corner of my healing room. Now, here was a cat thousands of miles away in the United States chasing the 'lump of black meat'. Cats do not normally go chasing nothing, but they will sometimes chase a ball or a similar object and paw at it with their front paws as this one was obviously doing. Feline Aids, or a lump of black meat, perhaps mistaken for a ball or some other such plaything for it to chase. An amazing performance I am sure you will agree. But there was more to come.

As the cat's owner regained her composure after the initial shock of seeing the cats reaction she realised that there would be more negative energy to clear, so she picked it up and put it back on the table again. Sure enough, there was still a lot of pressure building up between her hands again, but she decided she would not throw it over there again for the cat to chase as it had done the first time. This time she turned to her right and threw the unwanted dross in the opposite direction to where she had thrown the first lot. But this was one very smart cat she was dealing with and it obviously had no intention of being fooled that easily. It merely jumped off the table and chased this new 'ball' into the other corner. Is it any wonder that when medical people tell me that what I say I do is all in my imagination and they could never believe I could possibly do anything by waving by hands over a body. I feel like remarking that the animals must be far more clever than they are. Perhaps our animals have not been brainwashed into believing that their way is the only way. That anything else is so far outside the traditional boundaries of science that it is not even worth giving any consideration to it.

Sunday 9th August had been a rewarding day with one class from 9:30 am to 12:30, followed by a similar one after lunch from 2 to 5, while Monday was a complete copy of the previous day. As there was an average of around 20 in each of these four classes, the total number of students for the two days just topped the 80 mark. But at the end of each of the workshops they were told that as I would not be driven to Florence in Massachusetts until Tuesday afternoon, anyone who was free on Tuesday morning would be welcome to come back to Lisa's and we would set up several couches so that they could have healing if they needed it. While I say, have healing, I am not referring to me giving them healing. This was to be a practise day for all the really keen students who wanted to learn that little bit more which would set their feet on a firm path towards becoming efficient Magnetic Healers.

I had no idea how many of the original eighty would make the effort to attend a second session, and of course I was well aware that as this was a Tuesday, many of them could be expected to be working. As the time approached for the start of this get together I was more than thrilled to see one car after another pulling up in front of the house, while a number of the occupants were displaying their keenness to participate by carrying in a folding healing couch to set up in this large room. It was not long before I was able to count a total of 50 very keen would be healers filling the room plus a few who were gathered around one table in an adjoining room. The photo on page **124** shows at least 27 of these gathered around two or three of the couches. Some are healing, some are watching. But all are learning, and as the morning wore on and positions were changed, most of them had a chance to become the patient on one or other of the couches, while all were given the opportunity to participate as healers working on several different patients in order to be able to feel the negativity in different areas on the various patients.

Perhaps in one sense, this particular morning had to be the highlight of my whole trip to US, I had spent two very busy and quite tiring days showing these people what Magnetic Healing was all about and trying to get through to them that they, too, could be used as channels for his healing energy if their desire to be of service to their fellowman was deep enough. And now, here on the third day, I could stand back and reap the reward for my efforts. Here was a group of people who only a day or two ago had no idea they could be used in this way, yet here they were with me taking no more than a supervising roll in the whole proceedings, lining up at one or other of the couches to prove to themselves that they were now quite capable of finding the source of a problem in an ailing body and working to remove it. I slept well that night as I contemplated the long-term result of my efforts as at least some of these students continued to make use of their new found ability to heal their fellowman in need in the months and years to follow.

11. MEASURING THE ENERGY

If you take a careful look at the photo which shows the group in Vermont practicing on my last day there, you will see there is a lady wearing a red top working over the leg of the patient, but there is also a man in a white shirt who is doing something quite different. He is holding a metal object called an Aurameter which he is using to detect any negative energy in the aura of the patient. This is an extremely accurate and effective method of diagnosing, or if you wish, divining, to find out exactly where the source of a problem is in an ailing body. For me to explain how I came to discover this very efficient instrument, I have to take you back to England in 1997 where I stayed with my friend in Bristol as mentioned in Chapter 8. While he did much of his divining for water and energy fields in the many ancient areas such as Stonehenge and Avesbury with L wires, one day he brought out something I had never seen before. On inquiry I found that it was called an Aurameter and that he had imported it into England from where it was made in Santa Barbara, California, USA.

I was really intrigued by this instrument, and could immediately see that it held great possibilities for the accurate diagnosis of any problems in a body. I have always said, right from the time I first began to run my hands through the energy field of a body, that the only place a healer needs to worry about is the source of the problem. I cannot stress too strongly the importance of recognising this simple fact. I had seen healers such as Reiki practitioners placing their hands on the shoulders of a patient and I would think to myself why are they putting their hands there. I knew there was no problem in the shoulders so I could see no reason for placing their hands there other than the fact that as part of their training they had been told to do this. Just why I have not discovered, but for me I still say the only place a healer needs to put his or her hands is where there is a group of cells which has become out of phase and consequently is causing the body to be unwell in some way.

Would a mechanic use both his time and his energy to work on the carburettor of a car if he was aware that the problem he was supposed to repair was an electrical one? I am sure you would agree that he would not do that, yet I see healers doing what to me would be the equivalent of doing so, placing hands on shoulders or some other place their instructor has told them they should put them when the problem the patient is suffering from is located in the stomach or some other area which has nothing in common with the shoulders whatsoever. Maybe I was just born dumb or something, but I am afraid my mind has difficulty in trying to fathom out why anyone would do that when they should be going directly to the source of the problem to work there to restore the cells which have become out of phase with the rest of the cells which go to make up the body.

While I do not need to use an Aurameter, and in fact had worked on several thousand bodies before I saw the first one in Bristol, I have found it to be a very useful instrument. This applies particularly to my work as a teacher. When a patient is laying on a couch in front of a group of students I can use it for visual effect. If the patient has blood which is full of poison perhaps as the result of a malfunctioning liver, then I will demonstrate to my students that it is quite difficult for me to move my hand along above the leg because of the amount of resistance to its progress. If I pick up an Aurameter and hold it in balance above the foot of the patient, then move it along toward the knee, the pointer of the instrument will refuse to go forward and will lag back toward the foot as I move my hand and the handle forward. If there is nothing wrong with the blood, then the pointer will remain straight in front of the handle and move along the leg as I take my hand forward.

Having shown the students that there is a lot of negative energy in the blood by the way the pointer is refusing to move along the artery I then ask the first student to come up and remove some of that negative energy by cupping it away with his hands. If the blood is really bad I may ask two or three of them to come up and take some of it away but asking them not to move their hands along any further than the knee. My next move is to pick up the Aurameter and start again at the foot as I did before the students worked to clear the aura. Having already seen that the pointer had refused to move along the leg, they can become quite excited when they see it now moving along without any problems. I praise them for having done such a good job of clearing the negative energy in the patient's aura, and then continue to move it further along. As it reaches the knee it once again refuses to go any further and the students can see for themselves that while they have cleared the aura as far as the knee, the rest of it is still in the same bad state as the lower half of the leg was before they worked on it. I find it is this positive visual proof which goes such a long way towards convincing them that there is no doubt that they are quite capable of removing negative energy from a patients aura and by so doing bring new health, hope and upliftment to their patient.

When I hear a patient who has just walked out my door onto the concrete path saying to me that they are so light that they feel as if they are floating above the path, then I know that my hand and the Aurameter if I have used it, has without doubt divined the source of the patients problem and that at least a large portion of that problem has been removed. At this time as I pen the words, for this chapter I have titled "measuring the energy" I feel that in many respects, for a lot of my readers, this will be the most important chapter of them all. It is the one which is designed to help you to understand what Magnetic Healing is all about, and the vital difference between working on a physical level as orthodox people do, and working through the higher frequency energies which surround that physical body. The physical level consists of a low frequency vibration energy which is very limited in its ability to help the practitioner to discover the real source of a problem in a body. But the moment you step up to those higher frequency energies, the life-force which surrounds it, you immediately supersede all of those limits and the finding of that vital source of the problem becomes a simple matter.

Just as the little Maori girl mentioned in an earlier chapter was being scanned for any problem in the brain which may have been causing her to have up to six or seven epileptic fits in a day, so I find many others are being tested for all sorts of problems, but as in her case they are looking in the wrong place. If only her doctor could have understood that all he needed to do to find the source of the problem was to run his hands through her aura or use an Aurameter which would have refused to move past the female area, he would have known immediately that the real source of her epilepsy was a simple hormone imbalance which in turn was affecting the brain and creating the fits. But there is no way he would have been able to help her by scanning the brain as he had been doing, simply because there was nothing wrong there other than the fact that it was coming under too much stress from the hormone malfunction.

How long is it going to take us to get through the barrier which orthodox science and medical people insist on maintaining around them to the detriment of suffering humanity who deserve better than to be told that they think their problem is just stress as I have been told by so many desperate patients who have come to my healing room as a last resort when all else has failed. When will they ever learn that everything in a physical body is reflected in the life-force which surrounds it, and with this understanding will come the ability to leave behind all the guesswork which they so depend upon in the average doctors surgery today, and discover that the true source of the problem can be found by the use of a hand, or even more conclusively, an Aurameter. It should be realised that by using this method it is not possible to work in the wrong place on a body, simply because nothing will happen where all the cells are in perfect balance. The only place your hand or the Aurameter will react in any way is immediately above the group of cells which has become out of phase and is therefore creating a negative area in an otherwise positively vibrating auric field.

Being a very simple man, let me use some of that simplicity in an attempt to explain to you how a healer is able to guarantee that he is working on the correct area of a body, and not on some place where there is nothing wrong. There is a good reason why I have called what I do, Magnetic Healing. We all know enough about a magnet to know that the molecules of the metal have been especially aligned in one direction in order to create a field around it. We can prove this by bringing another magnet close to the first one. Like poles repel, unlike poles attract. In other words, if the positive ends or the negative ends of two magnets are brought together, they will push each other away, while a negative and a positive end will be drawn together. Let us consider for a moment a very ordinary looking wooden table about six feet long, you are standing beside it holding a magnet in one hand. You move this hand along, above the table, and as you expect absolutely nothing happens. There is no reason why anything unusual should take place. A magnet and wood have nothing whatsoever in common so you would not expect any response.

But after a while you move your hand much further along the table, and as it approaches about three quarters of the way to the other end, you suddenly find that your hand does not want to move any further. It is as though it has come up against a barrier of some kind and you are at a loss to understand why this should be when the wooden table looks exactly the same in this area as it does over the whole surface. The secret lies in the fact that unbeknown to you, someone has screwed a magnet underneath the table top precisely beneath the area where your hand is now feeling like it is being drawn in to that one spot and does not want to move away without you having to use some force to break it away.

Just try to visualise this scene in your minds eye, then bring that analogy to your healing couch. The table which your hand was moving along becomes the body of your patient. You do not know it yet but this patient has just one problem, and that is in the area of the heart. Unlike the doctor in his surgery who has questioned the patient to discover why she has come to his surgery, you have been told nothing of her reason for visiting you and neither do you need to be. As your hand moves along the body you feel nothing. This time of course you are not holding a magnet in your hand. You do not need to, because around your hand is an energy field, a part of the aura which surrounds every part of your body. Every cell is in perfect working order, so each one is surrounded, by a positive field, then like the two magnets which are brought together with like poles facing each other, your hand and the patients body beneath it will tend to be kept apart.

But as you approach the three quarter mark as you did on the bare wooden table, something quite different takes place, your hand suddenly refuses to move any further and you are aware that there is something quite different about your patients aura in this particular aura. And what is that difference? In this area a group of cells has changed polarity. Instead of being positive like all the others, this group has become negative, or as I often put it, they have become out of phase with all the rest of the cells which go to make up that body. So now we have a positive field around your hand approaching a negative one. As we have said, unlike poles attract, and so your hand is now being drawn into that particular area and you find that you cannot move your hand past it due to the resistance created by the law of unlike poles attracting. Your patient has still told you nothing, but you are already aware that this is the precise area where she has a problem, and so without questioning her in any way, you now know why she has come to visit you.

There can be no guesswork on a couch where one is practicing Magnetic Healing. The only place where you feel the resistance to the movement of your hand is the area where your patient is suffering from some problems. The question I am asked so many times is whether this healing can be of any help for a particular problem. Sometimes the name they give me is some long medical name I can hardly pronounce, leave alone spell, but my answer is always the same. For me, and I think I may have already stated this somewhere, there are no different problems. I leave doctors to put names on whatever has gone wrong with his patient. For me there are only cells which are in perfect working order, or cells which have broken down for some reason and become negative or out of phase. If every cell in the body is in good working order, then your hand will move from one end of the body to the other without coming up against any resistance whatsoever.

But if it stops somewhere and refuses to move any further without using a considerable amount of force, then you will know that your hand has now reached the place where you need to apply the healing energy to restore them to become positive again and the body at ease instead of diseased.

I do hope this explanation has not been too simple for you to understand. If you are an ordinary average simple down to earth person like myself, then I feel sure that understanding something so basic will create no problems for you, but if you happen to have been highly educated in the accepted scientific manner then I realise you may need to go through it again in order to figure out how anything so important as bringing new health to an ailing body could possibly be as simple as the above explanation. It may seem strange to you that I would suggest that someone who has been given a lot of education may find the above more difficult to understand than someone who has had no more than the basic schooling we all have before going on to a University or maybe a school of Medicine. But many years of experience has taught me that years of learning at such institutions can do little more than continue to perpetuate the beliefs your teachers had hammered into them by a previous generation of teachers when they were in your place. For me, it is now 67 years since I left school as a twelve year old boy with a school leaving certificate, but I am well aware that the School of Life I have been attending through all those years has taught me far more than I could have ever learnt in any University.

Don't get me wrong. Don't think for one moment that I am suggesting that you should not go to a University if you have the opportunity to do so. What I am saying is that you should be prepared to question what you are taught and ask yourself whether there is any proof that this statement or that particular reasoning can be accepted as the whole truth and nothing but the truth as they may say in a court of law. Remember that the only thing with any real value is truth, and you will find so much of what we are told through our media is just so far from it that you will very soon discover that you have been deliberately led away from it in an attempt to coerce you into believing just what they want you to believe. For instance, if you were at the head of a very large and profitable drug company, and you suddenly discovered that you were losing a lot of sales, and therefore a lot of your profit, simply because many people were being healed by other methods which did not use drugs at all, what would you do about it. Would you just let it carry on and continue to lose your profits, or would you do something to discredit this other method so that the people would go back to the doctors and have prescriptions written out again? Experience has told me that is exactly what they do.

In the instruction book which the makers of the Aurameter produce, the author makes the following statement. "Since it is forbidden in the US under Federal and State laws for anyone but a properly licensed doctor to diagnosis and treat a sick patient, no more will be said here, except that ordained Priests, Ministers and other members of the clergy can, within certain limits, participate in Spiritual healings through the application of prayer and laying on of hands. The Aurameter is definitely not to be used in any kind of diagnosis, treatment, or healing work".

I find this to be a very interesting statement, and one which calls for some degree of comment. It can be seen from the first part of that quote, that the American Medical Association has obviously done a very good job of protecting its members by having laws drawn up to ensure that no one else is able to find a problem in a sick body and do anything to help that person. I think this is called monopoly, and is obviously designed to ensure that any money available for helping people who are ill goes in one direction only. I see this as having little to do with sympathy for sick and suffering mankind, but everything to do with the mighty dollar.

As for the last sentence, where the author states that the Aurameter is definitely not to be used in any kind of diagnosis, treatment or healing work, I can only imagine that this has been placed there to protect his business from being targeted by the above mentioned associations, and I cannot blame him for being wise enough to do this. Big business will stop at nothing if they think that someone is undermining their monopoly, so for him to suggest that people buy his Aurameters so that they can use them to diagnose problem areas in their friends could be tantamount to committing suicide. Of course, at the same time, if we look carefully at this situation, it is not difficult to see that there would be little point in having them for sale and people buying them if those buyers had no intention of using them. While I agree there are a number of other uses which they can be put to, from my experience after selling a number of them to students, I have rarely seen them used for other than, I was going to say, diagnosing the sick but perhaps I should be a little more careful and change that to divining on the premise that doctors diagnose a problem in the physical body of their patient, while healers divine for negative areas in the energy field which surrounds it.

I would like at this point to ask you to go back and read that last sentence again before going any further. I have a feeling it is probably one of the most important sentences I will write in this book. So do read it again and think carefully about what it states. We are talking about two very different things here all in the one sentence and this is the distinction which I want to make quite clear to those on both sides. It is necessary to attempt to get through to those in the medical world that a Magnetic Healer is not working on the physical as he is. While the hand may at times come down close enough to the body to touch it, as no clothes are removed it is seldom that a hand touches the actual skin of the patient at all. Unlike the doctor who may press and probe, and push some instrument into one or other of the various cavities, or even use a gloved hand, the Magnetic Healer needs to do none of these things. He or she is not working on that physical body as the doctor is. We are working through that Life-force energy, the aura, which surrounds it.

If everything within the physical is reflected in duplicate in the energy counterpart then why would you need to probe the physical and cause distress, discomfort and embarrassment to the patient, particularly when that patient happens to be of the opposite sex to the practitioner. I can tell you now that is not necessary at all. Working through the energy field not only eliminates all of those problems I have just mentioned, but is also totally painless for the patient, takes less time, needs no expensive equipment and most important of all, is infinitely more accurate. If you think that claim is a bit wild, then all I can say is, I just wish it was possible for me to pass in front of your eyes and your ears a panorama of the thousands of cases I have attended to in the last thirty years where my patient has described to me some of the embarrassing situations they have been through. Some of them have suffered these indecencies a number of times over a long period of time, in the doctor's surgery and even more so, in the hospital they have been sent in to in an attempt to find the source of their problems.

And to think, that if only the doctor had learned to use his hand as a divining instrument, or even better, for more accuracy, an Aurameter, all of that could have been avoided. He would have quickly and accurately discovered that all important SOURCE of that problem, without even touching the body. Perhaps then, he could have even been able to follow in the footsteps of his great father of medicine, Hippocrates, and pulled and drawn away from his patient the aches and diverse impurities from which his patient was suffering. And again I ask you to view the panorama. And what do we see this time. We see some of the many frightened little children which have been brought to my healing room by their parents. We see them all too often, kicking and screaming, and if they are old enough assuring us in no uncertain terms that they do not want to be put on my couch. These are ones who have already been on all too many couches before. They have been pricked and probed, and jabbed with needles and there is no way they want to go through that again. Unfortunately, many times in such cases, in spite of all the reassuring by both the parents and myself, I can be half way or more through the whole session before it finally dawns on them that we really are telling the truth, and I am not about to jab them with yet another needle. It can be so rewarding to see as I have seen so many times, a scared and screaming child, spending the last part of his time on my couch smiling and questioning me as to why I am doing this or doing that, and obviously in no great hurry to get off the couch.

Why then, would any organisation want to take someone to court for doing what I have just described to you? I make no secret of the fact that since discovering that first Aurameter in Bristol, I have used one to "DIVINE" the negative energy immediately above the area in a body where the cells have become out of phase many times, and I can assure you that I receive many cards, letters or phone calls from grateful patients thanking me for having finally discovered the source of their problem and been able to do something about removing that problem for them when orthodox medicine had totally failed to even find what was creating the trouble. How much longer will it be before the world wakes up to what the great Nicola Tesla was talking about when he told us that in that single decade when science first begins to investigate the <u>non-physical</u>, they will make more progress in that decade than they have made in the past Century. How quickly we will supersede all the present limits we labour under by working on that very low frequency vibration of energy which we call the physical body, and step up to the higher frequencies which surround it. The Aurameter of course, has many other uses apart from finding the source of the problem in an ailing body, so for those of you who may be interested in learning a little more about energy I will mention a few of them here for you. After all, I have titled this chapter 'Measuring the Energy', so I guess this should be the appropriate place to discuss the measuring of any energy. Anyone who has attended one of my meetings, no matter where it may have been in the world, will almost certainly have heard me make the following statement. "For me there is nothing else in the whole Universe but energy. Energy in its many forms and frequencies of vibration". Everything we see with our very slow eye-brain combination we only perceive because those items happen to be made up of atoms vibrating slowly enough to allow us to detect them. And so we say to ourselves, this object, be it another body, a chair, a tree or whatever, is what we call solid matter.

But of course, there is really no such thing as solid matter. There are only atoms with spaces in between, infinitesimal as the spaces may be. There is so little we know about the properties of energy that there will be very little I will be able to tell you about 'why' those things which I am about to mention here actually take place. What I do know through many experiments is that they do. And are repeatable at any time in any place. While I was busy writing this page this afternoon, my telephone rang. On the other end was a very distressed man who lives in a small town about 150 miles south of my home. He was ringing to ask me if I would give him some absent healing and to see if I could find the source of his problem which was really getting him down. I stood beside my couch where I had placed a small piece of paper with his name and address on it, then asked for this one to be placed before me. I placed my right hand where his left foot would be if he was there in the physical form, and told myself that all I wanted to do at this stage was to clear the blood from the foot right along the leg and up as far as the heart.

I was actually surprised to find that nothing was happening as my hand moved along above the couch. I expected he would most probably have a lot of poison of some sort in his blood, and possibly have a malfunctioning liver after what he had told me concerning his condition. But even after all my years of healing, I can never be sure at this stage. The only thing I can be sure of is what my hand tells me, or if I am using it, the Aurameter or Energy Check as I often call them. After running my hand carefully, first from one foot and then the other up to the heart, I had to admit my guess had been totally wrong as the blood turned out to be in very good order and there was nothing there which either the hand or the Aurameter was able to detect.

I now took my right hand back to his left foot and suggested that it would now discover any other negative energy as I moved it up the leg. Its movement was quite free as I took it along first one leg, and then the other, so this told me that everything in that area was in good working order. Now came the torso, and as my hand came up the centre of the couch and approached the area where I visualised the base of the torso to be, it came up against a resistance which would have been about equal to pushing my hand against the wall behind me. As this was the centre of the body where the male organs are situated I immediately got the impression that like the little girl I had healed on TV, this was another one of those hormone problems which I all too often find myself faced with.

At this stage I picked up an Energy Check and began moving it up the centre of the couch. As I had expected there was no way that it was going to pass that area where the hormone problem had stopped my hand. I called out to my wife and asked her to bring my camera and to take a shot of what was happening. Thanks to the 'coincidence' of this man ringing me just at the time I was writing about measuring the energy with an Energy Check, we now have for you the photo on page 125 which shows you very clearly what happens when you ask for a certain person to be placed on the couch in front of you and then proceed to divine for any negative energy which may prove to you exactly where the source of the problem lies in that body.

While I am aware that because I do not have Doctor in front of my name and do not have several letters after it, there will be few scientifically trained people who will bother to read this book, but if there should be one who feels that he or she can give me an explanation of just how it is possible to detect negative energy in a body many miles away, and to be able to ring them up and tell them about the source of their problem I would be very grateful if that one would contact me and explain this phenomena to me. I must admit I really do not know how this is possible, but what I do know is that it does work, and very well at that. And may I add in all sincerity that if there is one out there who doubts my integrity in this matter and feels that he or she already "Knows" that this is impossible, then I will be anxiously awaiting that ones phone call or letter.

I would be very happy to set up an experiment to be carried out at some place of mutual convenience, where I would be given the name of some sick person who would like me to give them healing, and I will place that ones etheric counterpart on a table and then tell the doubter exactly where the problem is in their friends body. They do say that seeing is believing, but I am afraid that years of experience has taught me that there are none so blind as those who do not wish to see, so I will not hold my breath while I await that call lest I run out of breath long before it eventuates.

While I appreciate that anyone who has been trained in orthodox science would find it extremely difficult to accept that the above experiment really does work, I am well aware that there are many other quite amazing things which can be done by the use of the Aurameter or Energy Check which these same people would find to be equally as difficult to believe. So let us take a look at one or two of them, because I know there will be many more fortunate readers who will find these experiments both interesting and enlightening. Before someone starts wondering why I used the words 'more fortunate', I had better explain that what I meant was, people who still have an open mind. Remember the parachute and the saying, 'Minds are like parachutes, they only function when they are open'. These are the fortunate ones I am speaking about. The ones whose minds have not been closed off to everything except what they have been taught and told was the only truth.

Another photo on page **125** shows the pointer of the Energy Check lifting away from above a photo of the Crop Circle I found in Shrewsbury in 1997. You may remember that I actually found this Crop Circle by using a different devise for divining the energy which had been used to bend the wheat in the first place. Perhaps it is bad enough for some readers for me to suggest that there was enough energy left in that circle the day after it was made for me to be able to pick it up with the L wires from the best part of half a mile away. But when I tell you that every photo of a Crop Circle carries with it some of that energy which was used to make it, you may well consider I am going too far with that statement. If this is so then that will be no skin off nose as they say, but it will be you who will be the loser by refusing to accept something which you can prove for yourself if you wish to do so.

Of course the photo I took in Shrewsbury is not the only one the Energy Check works over. I have a large sheet of paper with eight colour photos of different Crop Circles on it, and I have found that it would appear that the actual shape of the Crop Circle has a bearing on what the Energy Check will do if it is held over any one of these. If the pointer is held above one photo, it will bob up and down for as long as it is held there, but if you move it across to the next one the bobbing may well cease, and the pointer will begin to fly back and forth from one side of the Crop Circle to the other.

While I have been using the words Crop Circle here, I should point out that I am not necessarily speaking of circles at all. Many of these are what are more commonly called Pictograms and can be any one of many beautiful shapes and as much as several hundred feet long. But whatever the shape or the size, I again challenge any scientist to explain to me why and how all this happens. And do remember that by turning your back on it all so that you will not have to look at it in case such happenings should be contrary to everything which you have been taught, and would be well outside the traditional boundaries of science, will not stop it from happening. These things of which I write here are as sure and as real for all to see if they so wish, as the sun rising tomorrow or setting at the end of the day.

But dare I write here of other experiments which in their seeming impossibility go far beyond anything I have yet recorded. I have already mentioned how I call the etheric counterpart of an ailing body onto my couch and work on that one even though they may be on the other side of the world, and have produced a photo for you of the Aurameter or Energy Check recording the negative energy of a patient some 150 miles away. But if I were to tell you that it is also quite easy to measure with the same very sensitive instrument, the energy of the body of one who has long since passed on and left that physical body, then I suppose I can hardly blame you if you insist on drawing the line at this point. This is a simple experiment I have conducted a number of times in halls full of people in several countries, and it has never failed to work so far.

To do this I simply stand in front of the people holding the Energy Check in my hand with the pointer facing away from me and wait for it to settle down so that there is no movement whatsoever. I then ask for all the people in the hall to visualise a photograph of the late Mother Teresa immediately in front of the pointer, and to hold that thought in their minds. I tell them that the fact that Mother Teresa is no longer on the Earth plane will have no bearing on the success of this experiment. It is not the physical body we knew as Mother Teresa which we are measuring. That low frequency physical energy has ceased to exist and we are measuring the higher frequency life-force which animated that body while it was on the Earth plane and gave it what we call life. When that energy was withdrawn and the body began its journey back to the dust from which it came, just as all humans do, that life force continued to exist, and this is what we are measuring.

As I stand there holding the Energy Check, it is not long before the pointer begins to respond to the energy of the thought pattern which all the people in the hall including myself are putting out, and it begins to bob up and down. But always with Mother Teresa it does not only bob up and down, but as it does so it also tends to go first to one side and then the other, continuing to rise and fall as it does so. I begin to feel a certain stress in my body and this tells me that the energy I am measuring has a dual personality of its own. The up and down motion brings with it a feeling of great love, yet as it begins to demonstrate the sideways motion I feel a tenseness which suggests a certain hardness mixed with that love. I remember reading an article written by someone who had once worked with Mother Teresa, and although she wrote about the great love of the one she worked for, she also mentioned that she was a very demanding and sometimes quite difficult taskmaster. I guess this would have been a part of her strong determination to get a job done and to allow no nonsense to get in her way in this regard. I feel it is this strong will of hers which I pick up in combination with the boundless love she had for her fellow beings.

I have been told that a thought pattern such as the people in the hall have produced can remain there for up to two hours, so I always like to move a few feet away before attempting to divine a different energy. Sometimes at this stage I will ask the people to think of the one we knew as Princess Diana, and to visualise her photo in front of the pointer of the Energy Check. It is interesting to feel the difference between these two energy fields. With Diana the pointer very soon begins to move in much the same up and down motion as it did when we first began to measure Mother Teresa's energy field. But there is one very noticeable difference here. The gentle bobbing up and down of the pointer in front of me continues for as long as I hold it there and we think of Princess Diana. There is none of the sideways motion. Just that gentle up and down movement and a peaceful loving feeling fills my body with no sign of stress whatsoever.

The age old fraternity known as the Rosicrucians obviously knew what they were talking about when they said that 'thoughts are things', and I believe this experiment goes a long way towards proving this to be true. On one occasion when I had finished the above experiment in a hall in a small NZ town, someone asked me if I had ever tried asking for a nasty sort of person to be placed in front of the Energy Check to see what difference there may be. As I had not thought of trying this, it was suggested that we try visualising a picture of Adolf Hitler. I lifted the instrument up and held it in front of me as usual, and it was not long before the pointer began to rise and fall. But this soon became something very different to the gentle motion we had just seen. It did not just move slowly up and down to a certain level and continue to do so as it had done with Diana. The up and down motion became violent as if it was attempting to get away from something it did not want to be near. It was not long before it was throwing back so rapidly that its backwards stroke began hitting me in the chest. But that was not the only reason why I decided to call it a day and bring the meter down beside me where it would no longer be facing what must have been a very powerful negative force field. The problem was that my breathing had changed and I had a strange feeling surging through my body. This was something I felt I could do without and immediately cut myself off from it as I dropped the meter down.

This experiment told me one sure truth as it confirmed for me that as a race of people climbing the long ladder of evolvement, we of Planet Earth know so little about the very basis of what we are, energy, that we must at this time be passing through the school of life at no more than the kindergarten level. What a long and painful journey we are going to have to travel through many incarnations if we insist on stubbornly refusing to lift our sights to higher levels of understanding. For as long as we consider ourselves to be physical beings, limited to those things which a physical being is capable of doing, then we can never raise our awareness of our true soul self within and come to understand that as living souls, sparks of God, limitless in our capacity as gods, we will remain forever chained to materialism and a continuance of the endless round of ignorance and fear which has carried us along the same old path of war and suffering for so long.

But this need not be. We can step away from this low frequency level of thought pattern and belief, and raise ourselves into a higher frequency level of vibration whereby we will become aware of our oneness with all that is, and the vast possibilities which lie within us waiting to be recognised.

Even though I have already conducted several hundred workshops wherever I have been around the world, I never tire of doing this. Mainly because each time I hold one I have the great pleasure of watching people who have up until that time, been tied as it were with chains to that low frequency level of belief, suddenly discover that they really do have this ability to be used as channels for the love force energy to flow to their fellow beings in need. It is not uncommon to see one break into tears or have to be helped back to their chair as the overwhelming truth of this discovery hits home. Just a few of the remarks which come from the lips of some of these give some idea of the effect this realisation brings with it. "Oh my God, it works for me". "Not my hands, but oh my arms". "Not my hands, but my tummy". "My whole body is tingling."

What we have tended to call 'common sense' tells us that this should not be so. We 'know' that this cannot happen. And when it does we can never be quite the same. There are some who will brush it aside and try to forget that it ever happened, simply because they feel they are not yet ready for such dramatic changes in their life. Fortunately there are others who immediately know within them that this is it, something inside of them says in no uncertain terms, this is the path I have been looking for. I always knew there had to be more, much more to life than the view I have had from the path which I have been following. These are the ones, who like the sceptic mentioned much earlier in this book, suddenly find that their depth of desire to be of service to their fellow beings is much deeper and stronger than they had ever imagined, and they set their sights on a life of service and dedicate themselves to be healers of body, mind and soul.

For some it is not even necessary to attend a healing class in order to see a light shining through what has been for them the darkness of ignorance and misunderstanding. Judging by the many wonderful letters which I have received from readers of my previous books, I am well aware that either the written word, or sometimes the spoken word, can trigger that something inside someone which tells them this is what they have been seeking, and this is the path they must follow. In keeping with what I always say about there being no such thing as a coincidence in my life, I received a letter this very morning from a lady about 360 miles from my home. Its contents tell me that while she would have no idea that I was busy writing my fifth book, it had to be much more than chance that she should write this letter at this particular time. An extract from it will cover beautifully what I have just written regarding the written word triggering something inside someone.

"Dear Colin, I have not finished your book yet. I am so excited I have to ask whether you are still teaching healing. I want to learn healing from you if you still teach. You may (and rightly so) believe that your book contains all I need to know. However, I would relish an opportunity to meet you in person. Your book is truly inspirational and I cannot believe I have not heard of you before. This is like finding the book I have wanted to read for years".

You may remember two things I have already written somewhere back there in this book. One concerned the number of people who have either written to me or phoned me to tell me they were half way through my wonderful book. Well here we go once again. "I have not finished your book yet". Familiar? And the other one was where I mentioned how so many use the word, inspire, or one of its derivatives. "Your book is truly inspirational".

And now as we approach the end of this chapter which was written in an attempt to bring to you some understanding of energy in its many forms and frequencies of vibration, and the methods which can be used to measure it and generally become aware of its existence, I want to point out to you some of the patterns which run through it. We have looked at the energy which surrounds a physical body, we have measured the energy which was responsible for animating several different physical bodies which have already passed the point of time which we so vaguely call death. We have also considered the energy created by Pyramids and Crop Circles. Now perhaps it is time to consider the written word.

What is the energy which is carried along far and wide with the words which I am now penning for your benefit. I can tell you that if I hold an Energy Check over a Bible, the vibration from the words it contains will start it gently rising and falling above it in very much the same way, and with that same feeling of love coursing through me that I mentioned I feel when I call on the energy of Princess Diana. Boundless love, unmistakable in its presence, and a joy to experience. If you look back at the words I just copied for you from today's letter, I think you will agree that words really can convey something which was built into them by the one who wrote them.

Just as the energy which was used to make the Crop Circles is still able to be measured even after a photo of it has been copied and printed in several thousand books, so it would seem that the energy which an author puts into writing words on paper in an effort to bring a new level of understanding and upliftment to his or her readers, continues to carry that energy no matter how many times it has been copied. The intent is there, and it would seem that nothing can remove it. I just pray that when the words I have written here find their way into the printing press, these words will carry with them a vibration which many readers will feel stirring within them just as the words which went to make up the book "You Too Can Heal" have obviously done for many readers including the one whose letter I received this morning.

12. WHERE TO NOW?

As we prepare to make our way into a new Millennium it is time for us to take stock of our situation concerning the health of the people of our planet, and to give very careful consideration to the path we should follow in this new and exciting time ahead. I say exciting, simply because that is the way I see it. The possibilities we are confronted with are enormous, but whether they become a help or a hindrance will depend entirely on what use we make of these possibilities. I hear people say there is no point in looking back at the past, because it has already gone so there is no way you can change it. That is a very true statement, but let us remember one thing. While looking back at the past will not change what happened back there, it can give us a guide to the future, and a very valuable one at that. None of us are perfect so we all make mistakes, but only a fool continues to make the same mistake over and over again, refusing to learn from them and stubbornly carrying on down the same old path which can only lead to the same result.

No one would dispute that Albert Einstein had a brilliant mind. His reasoning powers were surely much greater than the average human being, with the result that he made some very wise statements for us to ponder upon. But of all those statements the one I wish to quote to you stands out in my mind, as the most important that I have ever come across, not only from Einstein, but from any of the great philosophers. For me this extreme importance arises from the fact that the future of this planet and its people depends entirely on how we apply ourselves to the wisdom which is contained in it. If we ignore it, we lay ourselves open to everything from different levels of suffering and destruction to total annihilation. If we embrace it, and apply it with every ounce of effort we have available to us, then we open ourselves up to the possibility of raising ourselves and our environs to a level of which we have as yet barely dared to dream.

So let us look at his statement and we shall see whether you place as much importance on it as I do.

"The world we have made as a result of the level of thinking we have done thus far, created problems we cannot solve at the same level at which we created them".

So there it is. What do you think? Do you see it being as important as I do ? While I am not sure what date Einstein made this statement I presume it would have been some time after he emigrated to the United States in 1933. But whatever date it was, we can be sure that it would be even more true now than it was then. In the 1930's as a boy growing into teenage years I well remember the beautiful big peaches we had the pleasure of picking from two lovely trees my dad had planted, but what I do not remember is ever having seen him out there with a spray gun in his hand spraying poison on to the tree, nor do I recall ever hearing anyone mention a thing called an Ozone layer. There did not appear to be any necessity to concern ourselves with such problems, and of course these things are only the tip of the iceberg as far as pollution is concerned on planet earth and its atmosphere today.

There is one thing for sure, at the time of my boyhood, before this wonderful thing we have called "Science" held sway on the planet we would never have even dreamed that it would be possible for me to read a headline in a newspaper such as the following. "Cancer found in 10,000 veterans. More than 10,000 Vietnam war veterans in Australia have been diagnosed with cancer, according to official research which also raises deep concern about their children. New Zealand veterans anxiously waiting for the research findings have already been dismayed by an early disclosure of high rates of Spina Bifida among children of those surveyed. They have seized on this as further evidence of links between defoliants used in Vietnam, notably Agent Orange, and of birth defects in their own children."

Some of the figures which follow read like a horror story, but unfortunately they are the official records of the Vietnam Veterans Association. The list is too long for me to include here, but let me mention just a few to give some idea of the scale of the damage from this "Scientific breakthrough" as Agent Orange would no doubt have been hailed as when it was first manufactured. "Among the 25% of veterans who said they had been diagnosed with cancer, 405 had cancer of the colon – more than three times than expected, 137 with non–hodgkins lymphoma, almost triple the expected number, 64 with leukemia, twice as many as expected, and 51 with a very rare male breast cancer, more than 17 times that of the general population.

Those are merely the figures for the various types of cancer which have shown up, but of course there are many other problems such as 128 Motor Neuron cases, 138 of their children born with Down's syndrome, 50% more than normal, and 353 born with Spina Bifida, a whopping ten times the normal number expected. What I do find so difficult to understand is how the so–called scientists who spend their lives making big money inventing these death dealing formulas can ever manage to sleep peacefully again after they have read figures such as these. I am sure if I was responsible for having made it possible for these horrifying figures to exist at all, I would be having nightmares every time I closed my eyes and saw in my minds eye all those poor little suffering children with Spina Bifida alone, not to mention all the others.

Even in our "Clean and Green country" we are apparently not entirely guiltless in this sad story either. Evidence has been unearthed of a Government bid 31 years ago to supply NZ made chemical defoliants to US forces during the Vietnam war. While there is still no proof that they actually went there, it is quite clear the intent existed. Among the unearthed documents is a note by the late William Hutchings, then Secretary of Defence, recording the Taranaki companies interest in quadrupling its production of defoliants to supply US forces in Vietnam. The note was signed by both Mr Thomson Minister of Defence, and the late Sir John Marshall.

And what was the whole idea behind using thousands of gallons of defoliant to be poured down onto the forest from the air anyway. None other than to kill the forest. The very word they use for it tells us that. Defoliant. My dictionary says, defoliant, to deprive of leaves. So poor old mother earth was made to suffer again. We poured thousands of gallons on to her in order to strip the trees of their leaves so that there would be nowhere for the enemy to hide. Of course the hundreds of veterans and the many who have been suffering and dying like the forest ever since, just happen to be an unfortunate side effect of this wonderful scheme to destroy man and forest in one blow. Truly the wonders of science will never cease.

Is this the way we want to continue? As Einstein said, this is the world we have made as a result of the level of thinking we have done thus far. But do we really want to continue with that level of thinking and perpetuate these conditions for the generations yet to come? It may be too late for those who are already suffering from the effects and by–products of a diabolical totally negative science, but do remember that we can only bring change about by changing the level of our thinking pattern. We cannot solve these problems at the same level of thinking at which we created them was the way in which Einstein tried to show us what we must do.

If we are to survive as a race and continue to live a healthy life on the planet, then we MUST change that thinking. This low level vibration science must give way to a true science. The science of the higher frequencies as we move into a new dimension. While I do not like having to repeat myself too often, I feel that I must remind you here while we are examining the wisdom of Einstein and attempting to understand how we can put that wisdom into practise, that he was not the only one who could see that it was necessary for science to step aside from the path they were following and raise their thoughts to higher levels, moving from a science of destruction to one of construction. I am referring here of course to the statement I mentioned earlier where Nicola Tesla told us that in that single decade when science first begins to investigate the non-physical, they will make more progress than they have made in the past century.

And to what would he be referring when he speaks of the non-physical? Those of you who have read "You Too Can Heal" will remember the Kirlian photo I had produced on the front of the cover. It was a blown up picture of a finger tip showing the circle of glowing lifeforce around it, and in the middle I had written the words, "Energy, Key of the future" I have certainly not changed my thinking about that statement. While the orthodox medical fraternity still labours with the physical body in an attempt to diagnose the source of a problem in that body and decide which drug they should apply to it in an attempt to restore it to normality, the Magnetic Healer working through that high frequency energy, Tesla's non–physical, has already accurately divined the exact source and is drawing on the love force to apply it to those cells which have become out of phase. Surely it is not difficult to see what both Tesla and Einstein were trying to tell us when they said we must change the level of our thoughts to a higher frequency.

But unfortunately after all the years since these wise men made these incredibly important statements, science continues on its merry way seemingly oblivious of the fact that to continue to do so can only bring ever greater destruction and suffering for mankind. Why do they not learn from their mistakes? Consider for instance the newspaper I have in front of me at the moment. There is a large photograph of a man dressed in special clothing which totally covers him, head and all. He is driving a tractor between two rows of fruit trees and it is difficult to see much of the landscape around him because of a heavy mist. But this is not what we know as mist, tiny water droplets creating a fog which would be of little harm to anyone. The caption beneath the photo says, "Deadly Mist". It goes on to say that some sprays such as DDT, now known to be dangerous, were once hailed as marvellous discoveries and widely used.

And that is just the photograph and its caption, but the half page article has a very large headline saying, "Lethal leftovers in our blood", while the article itself points out that Dioxins are among the most virulent cancer causing chemicals. They go on to say that people over the age of 60 living in the Waikato, Bay of Plenty, Auckland and Northern regions are likely to have higher levels of Dioxin in their blood than other New Zealanders. I presume that for many people reading that article they would be learning something which they had not been aware of.

But that is certainly not true in my case. As one who has a healing clinic near the edge of the Bay of Plenty I have been attending patients for many years who have dragged themselves into my healing room and climbed onto the couch as if even getting there was an effort. In such cases, and there has been many of them, I almost always find great difficulty in moving my hand along the leg above the artery and I know that this is telling me that the blood in my patient has a very high level of poison of some kind in it, and I know I will need to work hard for some time to clear it for them.

But I am also aware that when I finally finish clearing the blood, my hand will then begin moving along the torso and will almost certainly be stopped in its movement as it approaches a badly damaged liver. At this stage I often say to the patient something like, "I'll bet you are dead beat tired". And nearly always the answer is in the affirmative. These ones are usually people who work in such places as Kiwifruit orchards where poison spray is an ongoing part of producing a "clean" crop of fruit to the detriment of the health of the workers. But pollution does not stop there. We read that the corpses of Atlantic sperm whales found along Germany's North Sea coasts contain such high concentrations of toxic pollutants that they should be classified as toxic waste says a study commissioned by Greenpeace. The Ecological Institute in Darmstadt, Southern Germany, found that the levels of some pollutants such as Polychlorinated Biphenyls (PCB.s) in the whales flesh and fat were too high for them even to be classified as sewage sludge. The examination showed that environmental pollution had reached an extreme extent even in the open Atlantic. The release into the environment of chemicals that are slow to degrade must be stopped as a matter of urgency. Unless that happens, survival of the big whales is seriously endangered.

Of course this sort of threat to the continuance of our existence on the planet is bad enough, but it pales into insignificance if you dare to take a look at something far more lethal which science managed to dream up. A news report tells us that nuclear experts worry about part of the worlds 3,000 tonne stockpile of bomb making material getting into the hands of rogue states or terrorists. For instance Russia's control over its weapons grade plutonium and uranium is far from airtight. They don't even know how much they have. Experts fear that a country like Iraq could steal even 200 grams of nuclear material and the Russians would not even know it was missing. It only takes a few kilograms of plutonium or highly enriched uranium to make a bomb. I ask you in all sincerity, if it only takes a few kilograms to make a bomb that could kill thousands, then what in the name of God are we doing with a stockpile of 3,000 tonnes? How many times do we want to be able to kill every man woman and child on the planet?

And just last week a news item had this to say. "Citing the risk of an accidental nuclear war, activists are pressing the US and Russia to take nuclear missiles off hair–trigger alert during the technology challenging year 2,000 rollover." They would like them to stand down the approximately 2,500 nuclear armed missiles now poised on each side for immediate firing. If Y2.K breakdowns produce inaccurate early warning data, or if communications and command channels are compromised, the combination of hair-trigger force postures and Y2K failures could be disastrous.

I realise that by the time this book I am now writing actually goes into print and you have the opportunity to read it, you will already know the answer to that dilemma. You will be doing one of two things. You will be breathing a sigh of relief that we made it through the difficult Y2K period and the buttons did not get pushed, or you will have joined the millions on the planet who will have returned to what I call the real world, the world of Spirit from whence you came when you entered your physical body, which like all the others, will have returned to the dust from which it came.

And to think that like so many others, I was until I read that article, naive enough to believe that the stories I heard so often about the "Cold War" being all over were actually true. How silly can we get. When will we learn that the very last thing they are ever likely to tell you is a thing called truth. If there is no cold war between US and Russia any more, why do they have to have 2,500 hair-trigger nuclear armed missiles facing each other. There is one thing for sure. If anything ever goes wrong here, that will be the end of the cold war, because it would immediately become the hottest war we could ever imagine.

The International Physicians for the prevention of nuclear war had this to say concerning a by-product of the gulf war. "It is not yet common knowledge that since the Gulf war the incidence of child leukemia has increased six fold, and there has been an increase in solid cancers in all age groups, particularly in Southern Iraq, plus an increased incidence of aids-like illness. This Is attributed to the use by the allies, particularly US and Britain, of depleted uranium as a by-product of nuclear weapons manufacture which is very dense. About 300 metric tonnes were used to increase the capacity of projectiles to penetrate, and for armour plating. On impact the uranium metal partially burns and generates large numbers of radioactive particles that are distributed in the dust. It is these particles, easily ingested or inhaled, that lead to an increased incidence of disease.

I am sure we have all heard the reference to the "Mad Scientist". I used to think that was something which was just said in jest, but the more I look at what is happening on our planet, the more I come to the conclusion that what I had previously thought to be a joke has become a horrible nightmare with no sign of it ending. And what about the disclosure just a short time ago that Britain's BSE - Mad Cow epidemic had cost the country four billion pounds, claimed the lives of 43 people and triggered fears that the death could reach several million. Some experts now believe it was caused by a "Scientific" experiment that went wrong. They believe hormones taken from the brains of slaughter house carcasses were injected into cows in a bid to create a new breed of super cattle.

But the experiment, done in the 1980's backfired. The hormones, extracted from the pituitary glands, were transmitted in an agent that spread Mad Cow disease and eventually infected humans as Creutzfeldt-Jakob disease. (CJD). "The theory is simple" says Dr Anne Maddocks, a retired senior medical scientist who specialised in infection control at St Mary's Hospital in London. "The promiscuous use of pituitary hormones in cattle led to BSE. in the same way that it led to CJD in humans. The timing of the death in cattle and humans who were exposed to pituitary hormones is very compelling." This was as much as I had intended to say about this particular subject, but a report in today's newspaper seems to be a fitting way of bringing this problem up to date with the latest information concerning the possibility of even more disastrous results from the original scientific experiment.

An enquiry has just been launched in London amid fears that the remains of slaughtered cattle at risk from Mad Cow disease could be contaminating the environment. The Sunday observer said the environment agency was urgently investigating the storage of 50,000 tonnes of rendered cattle carcasses in former aircraft hangars in Lincolnshire, Central England. The agency was forced to act after dead vermin were found inside one of the stores and gaps were seen in the walls of the buildings. The dumps should be airtight to prevent contaminated dust from escaping and being ingested by humans who might then risk contracting CJD, the human form of BSE. in animals. There are now more than 400,000 tonnes of the remains of cattle, slaughtered to eradicate BSE stored across Britain, and 80,000 tonnes of carcasses are being created each year. Because only one furnace in Britain is capable of burning the remains at 1,000 degrees C, the temperature necessary to kill the protein thought to transmit BSE to humans, most of the remains are stored in dumps.

That was some experiment wasn't it. Too bad it went so badly wrong. But of course, not even scientists would consider more experiments of a different kind which could harbour even a remote possibility of creating an even worse monster at some future time when it has already become too late to turn back the clock. Or would they? I am watching with a lot of interest and quite a large degree of concern, the continuing discussion concerning the experiments being carried out in many places including laboratories in our country, in an attempt to defeat nature by playing a game of monopoly with the very ingredients which go to make up every living thing on the planet. I refer of course to the mixing and controlling of the genes which determine what nature will provide in the way of food and nourishment for her offspring in every shape and form from plant to man.

It is not that many years since we became "Clever" enough to find out how to split the atom, the building blocks of nature, and we all know quite a lot about the disastrous side effects of that unforgivable mistake, from the tonnes of radioactive ash stored around the world from the generating plants, to the mass destruction of human life in Hiroshima and Nagasaki and on to the thousands of nuclear armed missiles waiting for the touch of a button which we talked about a little earlier. And now, once again it would seem that "Science" in it's ignorance and total disregard for the sanctity of nature is prepared to do battle with her again. Will they never learn that one thing they can never do, is to win that battle. She will always fight back in her effort to maintain the equilibrium which she knows is essential if her offspring are to continue to exist in harmony with her. But arrogance knows no bounds, and it will always be the innocent who will suffer for the transgressions of those who should have known better.

Already we have food on the shelves of our supermarkets which has been modified by what has become known as Genetic Engineering or GE. The whole history of Genetically Modified or GM food thus far has been one of giant corporates pushing the stuff into the market-place, just going ahead and doing it anyway, while governments and bureaucracies trail some distance behind, bleating about checks and balances. Always it seems, it is the power of the mighty dollar which controls our destiny, a path which has little to do with the welfare of the masses, but a great deal to do with the bank account of those corporates. It would seem that in this country the government reluctance to take a tough stand on GM foods stems from its fear of offending the US, home of the food technology giants such as Monsanto, and there is certainly a hint of that in leaked ministerial minutes from last year which refer to American concern that even a relatively toothless labelling regime could impact negatively on the bilateral trade relationship.

Monsanto released its first harvest of "Round-up-ready" soy beans on the US market in 1996 without labelling or segregation. Only a tiny percentage of Americans were aware of it. It was only when the company exported those same beans to Europe later that year and found the watchdogs known as Greenpeace waiting at the wharves in an attempt to stop the unloading that they received the first whiff of what was to come. To placate angry consumers, countries and companies were left scrambling to source non-modified soy beans themselves, an exercise which became a public fiasco.

Unlike conventional hybridisation, genetic engineering involves the transfer of foreign genes not previously present in a species gene pool. It can also cross the species barrier. This it is argued is more likely to have unpredictable effects on the consumer and the environment. If you were to ask me if I considered that the GM food which is already on the shelves of our supermarkets is any way harmful for us to eat, I would have to give you the same answer as Monsanto would have to give you if they were honest enough to say so. I would have to say, I do not know. And surely this is the whole crux of the matter. Nobody really knows for sure. I am quite prepared to agree that there is a good chance that it may well be quite safe for us to consume, but just like those who were responsible for the original splitting of the atom, we do not know what disastrous effects may turn up much further along the food chain.

It is not so much the fact of having some GM food on our shelves, but what I just mentioned about the possibility of the changes man has made crossing the species barrier and taking off into an uncontrollable nightmare of genetic misfits with disastrous results that really worries me. I can only hope that in a few years time I will not be writing book six which will contain details of those results. As one US based activist said, "If food producers are so proud of these 'Brave new world' products, then why are they so reluctant to label them". As we ponder the information contained in this chapter up to this point, we may well ask the question, "Where to now?

Surely the time has arrived for us to decide to what extent we are prepared to allow ourselves to be controlled against our will by an all powerful bureaucracy. But just before we do, for those of you who may be just a little vague concerning the meaning of that word bureaucracy, let us take a look at our Oxford dictionary and see what explanation they give. "Government by central administration. Officialdom. Red tape" There is more, but I am sure that will be enough for you to realise why I used that word long before I have finished the story which now follows. Unless you would like me to add the fact that the word 'Bureaucrat' is mentioned as one who is 'an inflexible or insensible administrator', and I think you may soon be agreeing with me when I say it is just such as these which we are about to discuss here.

In February of this year of '99 the NZ public suddenly found themselves eagerly watching the TV news broadcast or scanning the newspapers for the latest developments in a case which had suddenly hit the headlines with a force which one would have hardly have expected when you consider that it all centred on one little three year old boy known as Liam. It had been disclosed that the boy was suffering from cancer. He had a bump on his face and was being given chemotherapy in Dunedin Hospital for his Neuroblastoma. When his parents found he was not responding as they had hoped he would do, they decided that enough was enough and they would seek an alternative treatment. They said the decision to seek alternative treatment was made after much searching and real concern at the shortcomings of orthodox ways.

The family court authorised Healthcare Otago to continue chemotherapy and removed guardianship of the boy from his parents. The court appointed itself Liam's guardian and issued a warrant for police to hand him over to the youth agency after his parents failed to return him from a trip to Auckland in search of alternative cancer cures. It was Healthcare Otago that sought the family court's intervention, with doctors saying the boy had a

50/50 survival chance with chemotherapy but was likely to die in three to six months without it. His parents issued a statement in mid February saying his tumour was shrinking under alternative health care and that they had no option but to stay in hiding, given an uncompromising approach by Healthcare Otago. And so the search was on. As the "criminals" were sought wherever it was thought they may be hiding we were treated with pictures in the paper of police, as they put it, tightening the net and seizing papers showing the boy was treated at a Rotorua clinic.

One of the sixteen different articles I have concerning this case shows one policeman giving another a leg up so that he could peer over what looks like a garage door. The caption beneath the photo states, "Police search the Rainbow Health Clinic" in Rotorua for information about Liam's whereabouts." This was just one of several places they searched in an attempt to carry out the Family Court's order to bring the child in against the parents wishes so that Healthcare Otago could continue to give him more chemotherapy. What they did not know was the fact that my friend at that clinic had asked me to help the child by placing him on my couch and giving him what I have referred to as absent healing. This turned out to be quite an experience for me, as although the cancer was visible as a bump on his face, and I did work there, as so often happens in such cases, after spending some time clearing the blood, my hand was stopped on the lower right side of the torso.

Many times over the years when a mother has brought to me a child who is being treated for a brain tumour, I have found that I have worked much harder and longer usually somewhere around the lower torso area. I have long since realised it is very seldom that a child just has a brain tumour. For me this is almost always the secondary, and what my hand picks up in that lower torso area and I stagger away to the corner of the room with is the primary from which metastasis has taken place and the cancer cells have been carried to the brain where they have become lodged and set up this thing we refer to as a brain tumour. It was no great surprise to me to find that while working on a child who was suffering from a visible growth on his face, I found myself working so much harder and longer to remove a primary.

There was of course many letters to the editors of newspapers at this time, and a couple of them shown here will give my readers some idea of how the public reacted to the heavy handed treatment which was being handed out to the boy and his parents.

"It is appalling that in a free country (as NZ is presumed to be) people do not have the right to choose what they consider to be the most appropriate health care and treatment for themselves and their children. The case of young Liam made us aware of archaic attitudes and prejudices that still exist. The desire of his parents for a gentle return to good health for their son, instead of invasive experimental treatment with undesirable side effects, is to be commended. The response of the medical profession and their legal supporters is barbaric and belongs to a bygone era. People must have freedom of choice in all matters relating to the well-being of themselves and their children".

This second one was written in reply to a letter in a previous issue.

"According to Doctor Bill Morris, Western modern medicine provides the only valid kinds of treatment available for cancer. All equally valid forms of non-western medicine are conveniently lumped together in the categories of alternative or unconventional. Perhaps Dr Morris should apply some of his scepticism to his own profession. Examining the recent history of Western medicine, one looks back in horror at some of the crude forms of treatment (now invalidated by the medical profession itself) and wonder if soon chemotherapy will be added to the list. It is interesting to note how quickly doctors defend chemical companies over suggested links between the use of herbicides and pesticides and cancer. Perhaps the reason is that these same companies have in the past donated substantial sums to the cancer research."

Concerning the suggestion in the above letter that soon chemotherapy will be added to the list of crude forms of treatment, I have no doubt that the time will come when the beneficial use of energy is fully understood, people at that time will look back and say something like, "How did they ever allow the medical profession to use such a horrible chemical on human bodies with all the terrible side effects that it created? And believe me, I have heard many sad stories from patients on my couch over many years, and some of the worst of those concerned the hell they went through from those very side effects, with the loss of their hair being the most painless of them all.

By this time the parents, who wrote to a family friend, were saying that hiding from the authorities had not been easy. They were continually looking over their shoulder while they treated their boy with a portable electric pulse machine. And this is where I wonder whether perhaps they should have substituted the word 'authorities' with the word I used at the beginning of this story, 'bureaucracy'. Already I was having patients coming to my healing room from different areas of NZ who were almost without exception, becoming very angry and afraid. They would ask me questions which left no doubt in my mind that they were worried that something like this could happen to them if they had a child with cancer which they preferred to bring to me for healing rather than see the child suffer in the way that many do when they are being treated with chemotherapy.

In my third book, "Magnetic Healing and Other Realities" I told the story of the three and a half year old boy who had been carried into my healing room way back in 1981. At two and a half years of age he had developed leukemia, and for a full year he had been treated in the orthodox way which consisted mostly of giving him chemotherapy. After twelve months of this treatment the parents were informed by the oncologists at the hospital that they may as well take him home as there was no more they could do for him. Their actual words to the parents were, "We have done everything humanly possible. As you can see, he is now too weak to stand so you will have to carry him". This was two days before Christmas, so they suggested that at least they would have him home for Christmas as they expected he could live maybe a couple of weeks. He was brought to me from their home about sixty miles away on Christmas Eve and they were given the most wonderful Christmas present they could ever have hoped for as I spent a full hour working very hard to clear the leukemia from his blood.

It was a very surprised doctor who was confronted with the sight of the same boy trotting along beside his parents when they walked him into the hospital a few days later. But I am sure they would have been even more surprised if they could have had the pleasure as I did, of being a guest in a hall full of people when he celebrated his fifteenth birthday nearly twelve wonderful years later. He did finally pass away some time after that, but it was not due directly to the leukemia as they had his blood checked every six months and it never showed any sign of having returned. It is my belief that a year of filling up that little body with chemotherapy did so much damage to so many cells that the body finally just gave up. But as the mother said to me one day, "Colin, we had twelve wonderful years with our boy, and they told us that we could have no more than two or three weeks at the most."

It is cases like this which stir within me a desire to bring to the people the knowledge that there really are alternatives to the endless round of chemicals which a so-called science relies on in an attempt to balance the damaged cells of an ailing body. I still believe that the words, "Energy, Key of the Future" which I had written in the centre of a glowing orb of light around a

Kirlian photo of a fingertip on the cover of my last book will become recognised as exactly that, the key which will unlock the door to the future. The thirty thousand or more patients I have treated in my healing room and the thousands more I have had the pleasure and privilege of attending to in several other countries have left me with no doubt that this is the path which we must follow. This is the way we must go. If it was good enough for the great Hippocrates to 'pull and draw away aches and diverse impurities' with his hands, then it should be equally as effective for us today. Learn that there is nothing else in the whole universe but energy. Energy in its many forms and frequencies of vibration, waiting for us to recognise the endless possibilities which lie within our reach, when as Tesla said, science first begins to investigate the non-physical.

Learn to use the energy in a positive way and we will find that those things which we now refer to as miracles will become the norm and as the Bible says, the former things shall pass away. It is time to learn to go with nature and become one with her, instead of battling our way against her by poisoning everything from our bodies to the air we breathe, the land we need to give us sustenance, and the life giving water in our rivers and seas. When we can truly understand energy in its all pervading presence, then we will come to know that just as we should be using it to restore the damaged cells of a body, so we can use its endless existence to take us through the highways and byways of infinite space by drawing on it as others have obviously been doing at least since Job enquired as to who these were who flit from cloud to cloud and Ezekiel gave his wonderfully accurate description of what we now so vaguely describe as a UFO as he spoke of the wheel within a wheel with eyes all about.

It would seem that if we want to learn something new and beneficial for the good of mankind, then we need to look at the past and discover some of the knowledge which we have lost. From the burning at the stake by religious bigots of any who dared to show that they had been blessed with what Paul writes of in his letter to the members of the church in the City of Corinth as gifts of the Spirit etc, to the burning of the books of knowledge lest the ordinary people should gain that knowledge by reading them, our history is filled with the efforts of those who consider themselves as leaders, both religious and political, to retain their hold over the masses by keeping them in ignorance.

When you look back at what the leaders of our country did to Liam and his parents and the propaganda they put out to the rest of us to try to convince us that only they know what is best for us, I wonder just how much progress we have really made in this year of '99. And now as the double 9 is about to be replaced with the double 0 surely it is time for us to stand up and be counted. Time to say enough is enough, and to find the courage to speak out for our rights as citizens of a supposedly free world. It is time to have your say, and to demand that half-truths and innuendos be replaced by the powers that be by the whole truth and nothing but the truth.

It will not be an easy task to bring this about, mainly because in this day of the power of the mighty dollar, the drug barons and others who wield that power have no desire to lose their grip on the hold they have on you and I, the ordinary people who make up the great majority of the citizens of planet Earth. Control is their key word, and the penning of the sheep is their goal. As our world becomes ever more materialistic in its make up, with an ever greater desire by the masses for more and more material goods, so their ability to gain that hold continues to grow. We are the pawns in the game, to be moved and controlled as they wish. But it need not be so. Stand up for your rights and do your part in bringing about a brave new world of light and enlightenment where suppression will be superseded by equality.

Where to now? That depends on you. I know, you think there is nothing you can do to change it. But if we all think like that, then that is just exactly what they want you to do. You will be playing right into their hands. Complacency practised by the majority is all the few need to retain their hold over you and to be able to tell you what is good for you without you realising you are being told these things simply because they know that to have you accept them as truth is all they need for them to be able to perpetuate the control they already enjoy.

Earlier this evening while watching a programme on TV titled "The Supernatural", the compere who was talking about Crop Circles, assured us they were made by wind whirling around and bending the wheat in the shape of a circle. Does he really believe that, or has he been paid good money to try to fool us into believing that he is telling the truth. He stated that the circles are made by wind, and as if it was not of any great importance, sort of casually mentioned that the more complicated ones are hoaxes and not made by aliens as is popularly believed.

No mention of course of the fact that some of England's top engineers have stated that it would take them quite a long time to work out some of the very large Pictograms several hundred feet long, and that it would be almost impossible to produce them with such precision in the dark. And that covers most of them, because they nearly always appear over night. No mention either of the sort of energy they hold that allows someone to find one nearly half a mile away with a pair of L wires, not to mention the fact that when taken from a Crop Circle and tested in laboratories in Stroud, Gloucester, the energy pattern of the crystals produced by a distillation process showed a very different form to wheat from any other place.

I implore you at this crucial time in the evolution of Mother Earth and her children to keep your minds open and give some serious thought to the authenticity of the information which you are being fed. Do not accept everything you are told just because it is easier to do so than to use a little time and effort to find out whether it really is the truth. For of what use to you is a half-truth, leave alone some of the deliberate lies which are being handed out to us in an effort to hold the status quo. Remember, where we go to now will depend on you. Be sure to do your part in bringing about the brave new world of light and enlightenment.

13. BRIDGING THE GAP

In the first chapter of this book I mentioned how, over several years, as I watched so many students who had never felt negative energy in a patients aura before, place their hands over a body on the couch and suddenly find themselves coming under stress as they attempted to bring them together or to lift the problem away from the patient. At one stage I found myself saying to the group, "Look, Healers Unlimited". And they are, unlimited. They are everywhere. The only problem is, no one has ever told them so they do not know they have this wonderful ability laying dormant within them waiting to be recognised and used for the good of mankind.

And that is what I am really all about today. I do not claim to teach anyone how to heal. I simply become the catalyst which changes the beliefs, the thought pattern and the understanding of my students. I am not really adding anything to anyone. I am merely helping that one to recognise what has already been laying there dormant within, but unrecognised, simply because no one has ever told them it is there.

As I was writing that last line my telephone rang and my wife brought it in to me to answer. As I had not long sat down to start this last chapter I felt a little annoyed that once again I had been taken away from my writing just when I was getting into the swing of it. I should have known better, and realised there would be a very good reason for this interruption. And of course there was. On the other end of the line was a lady I had stayed with just two weeks ago about 250 miles south of my home. There had been the usual radio interview in the morning with a public meeting in a hall in the evening, followed by two workshops the next day. As usual, we had found that amongst the forty people who attended those two workshops there was a very large number of them who, for the first time in their life had discovered that very thing I have just been writing about. Their ability to be used as channels for the love force in search of peace and harmony and abundant health for their fellowman.

And why did she ring me? You probably guessed it. She rang to say that she thought I may like to know that two nights ago a number of those students had come together to have their first practise without my presence. Some students are a little afraid that they are feeling the negative energy at a class only because I am standing there helping them. They wonder whether they will still be able to do the same after I have left. It is this first occasion of getting together to try themselves out which I think some people feel a little afraid of. I am sure there are some in the group who would like to go along with the rest of them but feel they may look silly in front of the others if they come up to the couch and nothing happens when I am not there to guide them.

But as so often happens, my friend on the phone had rung to assure me that their meeting had gone off extremely well. When I asked her if everyone was happy with the results they had experienced, she said in simple words, "We were all wrapt". A strange word to use perhaps, but in this country anyway I think that almost anyone would translate that as meaning anything from very happy, to ecstatic.

Now what was I busy writing about when that phone rang? Oh yes, of course. I had just been saying something about helping people to discover their latent ability to heal laying dormant within them, and my part in helping them to discover it. And what was the phone call about? My organiser from just two weeks ago ringing to inform me that many of the group she had brought together in order for me to be able to help them to discover it were "Over the Moon" to find that they were now perfectly capable of becoming Magnetic Healers.

And so the proof keeps pouring in. Proof that there really is an unlimited number of people out there who could be using their hands and their hearts to bring new health to those in need. Their hearts you say. And I say again, yes, their hearts. Remember that most important of all statements I mentioned earlier. "That which you will achieve will be in direct proportion to the depth of your desire to serve". Surely this can only be found in your very heart of hearts, deep within your soul. A recognition of your true soul self within. The realisation that you are so much more than a physical being. These are the attributes which define one who is prepared to put aside some of the more worldly past times of ones normal life in order to make way for the use of your newly discovered abilities and to create the necessary spare time to be able to give them priority above the more mundane things of life.

Do remember, material things are always transient, of seeming importance for us today, and cast aside tomorrow. But you, that real you, was, is, and always shall be an eternal living soul, alternately incarnate and discarnate. Incarnate within the physical for a few short years, and discarnate once again when it is time for you to leave your very temporary home, and return from whence you came. And when you do, you will take with you the memory of all those things which you achieved while encased in that physical form, both good and bad. Your Karmic record will be added to on both sides of the page.

What do you want your record to look like at that time? Will the negative completely over ride the positive? Or will you be able to look back with satisfaction at those things which you achieved while you were on the earthplane.

I am often asked why I have spent so much time over many years spending endless hours either healing, lecturing, teaching or writing, when there were many other things I could have been doing if I so wished. I think to find the answer to that question, we need to go back 35 years or more, when like the students I showed the way of healing to just two weeks ago, I made a similar discovery to the one they have just made. As I felt the energy flowing through my hands and I began to realise that so much of what I had been taught up to that time had not been the simple truth I had been brought up to believe it to be, I somehow suddenly knew deep within that life for me could never be the same. I knew I had to find both the time and the desire to give of myself in abundance in order that those less fortunate could not only be helped in a physical sense by healing their bodies, but perhaps even more importantly, lifted up into new levels of Spiritual awareness and understanding.

Then came the evening when that most important message was given to me at a meeting after I had been doing some healing and someone said they would love to be able to heal bodies like that. "How great the healing of the body, but how much greater the healing of the soul." That was the message which was given to me, and I knew from that moment that it was time to get my priorities right and devote more time to those things which belong to the eternal part of man and less time and energy on the temporary. Some day it will be time for this short sojourn of mine on the earth-plane to come to a conclusion, and I will step aside from this physical form and return once again to that other level of existence. I would like to think that when I do so I will have earned the privilege of hearing those words which can be found within the pages of the book we know as the Bible, "Well done thy good and faithful servant."

Of course it is not for me to know whether anything I may have achieved at this physical level will have earned me the privilege of being given that recognition, but I simply strive on and do my best to attempt to make this possible. But more than that, my greatest hope is that through my teaching and my writing I will have been able to help to lead other souls onto the path of recognition which will give them the opportunity of maybe hearing those words spoken as they too reach the end of their time in the physical.

I have found in this work that life can be a little like riding on a roller-coaster. One can be up and down from a high to a low in a very short space of time. Let us go back for a moment to that little girl I worked on for the TV. Six or seven fits a day for eighteen months and never any sign of another one ever showing up after I worked on her. You could imagine that I would be on quite a high at this point, knowing that my time and effort was responsible for removing this distressing situation completely from a young child when the best medical help in the country had failed to even find the source of the problem, leave alone bring any relief to her whatsoever.

So here we are on a high spot, so why should there be any reason to find oneself suddenly dashed into despair. Unfortunately the answer to that question is all too simple. Buoyed by the flush of success I could see that there must be other children out there with a similar problem, so I reckoned that if I could just get through to the medical people the fact that they only needed to look at the hormone imbalance in these cases instead of scanning the brain for the source of the problem, then they should be able to bring new health to any patients who are brought to them with a similar problem.

But of course as you will have read earlier, that was not to be. The doctor assured me it was his drugs which were keeping her from having any more fits, in spite of the fact that they had done nothing for her over the previous nine months until the very day I had worked on her. And somewhere out there I knew there had to be other children I did not know about who would have to continue to suffer as our little Maori girl had done for nine long months just because minds are like parachutes, and they do not work when they are closed. Or are the real enemies here the twin barriers of ego and fear. Is it merely the fact that it is too difficult for one who has spent many years learning all there is to know about orthodox medical practises to accept that someone who has had no training along that path whatsoever, could suddenly cut the ground from under that ones feet by trying to show him a simple answer to a problem which with all his training he has failed to solve.

This is the ego side of the dilemma, but what about the fear. Could it be that the real opposition lies in the fact that they can see all too clearly what an acceptance of this simple yet so effective method of bringing new health to an ailing child, or adult for that matter, would mean to a Medical Association which is struggling to assure their customers, the sick and suffering, that the only people who can assist them are their members. Is it any wonder they make documentaries which are designed to show the viewers that alternative methods of healing do not work, and to tell them that if they visit one of those they will be missing out on what they could have had done for them if they had gone to a medical doctor instead.

Several years ago I first realised that there appeared to be little chance of breaking through the barrier which medical people seem to want to surround themselves with. I came to the conclusion that if they would not let me in through the front door to offer whatever I may be able to give to help in divining that vital source of a problem in an ailing body, then my only alternative was to go around the back and see if I could make my way through from there. While there have been a few open minded medics I have had the pleasure to work with such as the ones in Los Angeles and Vermont, these are very much in the minority. I felt that it was time to attempt to break through the barrier in order that so many who are missing out on the help which they could be receiving if the doctor was aware of that vital source would be able to enjoy the results which would follow.

So I finally came to the conclusion that if the few thousand patients one person was able to work on over a number of years was not enough to convince them to sit up and take notice, then maybe if there were many people doing this work they would begin to wonder why some of their usual customers were no longer visiting them. Hence the decision to go out and show others how easy it is to become a Magnetic Healer. I really have no idea how many groups of students I have worked with since that first class I took in Maui in 1987, but I do know that it would amount to several hundred.

I would love to be able to say that all of these people were continuing with the healing work, but unfortunately, that would be far from the truth. For reasons which I have already mentioned, there is only a small proportion from each of those hundreds of groups, but as you will have seen by some of the letters I quoted from which have been sent to me, usually, but not always, from the organiser of the group, there are quite a substantial number who are enjoying the success they are having. But more important, is the fact that some of these are now showing others what they have learnt. As they do this, so the overall number of practising healers is steadily growing.

One of those who has followed in my footsteps is a woman we know as Kathy. Kathy lives in a Central North Island City, and has been carrying on with the healing work for a few years now since I first showed her the simple technique. A couple of years ago we sat down to discuss the work and to bring together some ideas on how it could gain a little more publicity so that a greater number of people would know that there really are alternatives to the endless round of visits to the doctor and the inevitable pills etc. I mentioned to her that for some time I had been considering the idea of bringing together as many as possible of those of my students in NZ who were still continuing as healers. What I had in mind was just a loosely knit liaison between members so that they could visit each other if they were travelling, and by having a printed list of the names, addresses and phone numbers of all members, it would then be possible to direct people in need to those working in other areas.

Kathy decided she would make the effort to spend some time with her computer and organise such a group. By April of '99 she had not only done all the spade work to bring this about, but had of her own volition, organised a get together of all members who could manage to travel to Palmerston North where she had hired a hall for the weekend. This turned out to be a wonderful weekend for me. It was the culmination of untold hours of work, and many thousands of kilometres of travelling throughout the country. Friday was my day to be interviewed on the radio so that the people would know what was happening in their city over the weekend. Saturday was a day for the gathering together at the hall of the forty or more healers who had travelled from many different areas, while Sunday was set aside for the public to attend so that they could learn about this group of people who had come to their city under the name of "Healers Unlimited".

As you will see by the photos on page **126** I had the pleasure and privilege as founder of the group to give an opening address to all those gathered in the hall. Quite a few of the healers had brought their folding healing couches with them, and after my address these were set up along the centre of the hall. The public were then invited to lay on one of the ten couches, and experience, many of them for the first time, what it was like to have a Magnetic Healer working to clear the negative energy from their aura, and by so doing, bring new health to their body. As always happens, it was interesting to watch the faces of some of them as they lay on the couch and the healers hand stopped somewhere above the body.

A patient who has never been given healing like this before and is used to having to explain to their doctor where their problem is, can become quite overwhelmed when someone they have never seen before informs them that they must have a problem in a certain area because that is where his or her hand has stopped against some negative energy in their aura. Usually the patient is already aware of this, but he is also aware that the healer could have no idea that this was the very area where he was having pain or discomfort of some kind.

Some of us who were doing the healing would invite another member of the public to come up to the patient on the couch, and to place their hands over the patient in a position which we indicated as being the problem area. Most of these people had never even seen someone doing healing like this before, but when they began slowly bringing their hands together as we instructed them to do, some of them were blown away when they discovered a resistance which made it very difficult for them to bring their hands together. Having finally managed to do so and cupped their hands under the ball of negative energy, they were even more amazed to find that they were having difficulty in lifting their hands away from the patient. "It's too heavy, I can't lift it", are the words I have heard on a number of occasions when this has happened. But usually it needs to be something really serious in the body such as cancer before it becomes that difficult to lift it away. While I do not think we had any people on our couches that day who had problems of quite that order, there were many who did have enough negative energy in their aura to keep several healers busy for a large part of the afternoon.

For me, looking across that hall filled with my students from around the country, busily working to bring new health to all those people who kept on coming in all afternoon was a sight which, back in '87 when I held those first few classes in Maui, I hardly dared to dream I would ever see. Now at last I could begin to see the gap between orthodox medicine and alternative healing slowly closing as an ever increasing number of people discovered this method of healing really does work. And not only the fact that it does work, but also the realisation that so often it is not necessary to suffer all those nasty side effects from the many drugs and pills and potions which are the normal result of a visit to an orthodox doctor.

I still believe the time is rapidly approaching when orthodox and alternative treatment will merge and become one. This will be the time when the word alternative, will be exchanged for complementary. My Oxford dictionary tells me that 'complement' means one of a pair, or one of two things that go together. If we then look at 'complementary' we find this explanation. 'Completing, Complementing each other'. Sounds good to me. I could go along with that. But unfortunately up to this time the desire for complementing each other has been mainly one sided. Like many other 'Alternative' workers, I would like nothing better than to be able to 'Complement' the medical profession by working with them. But as you can see by what happened when I approached the doctor at our Starship Hospital concerning the little Maori girl with the epileptic fits, there was no way he even wanted to hear my explanation of the problem being created by a simple matter of hormone imbalance.

And again, if we return for a few moments to Liam and his parents who were sought by the police after the family court removed guardianship and gave it to the Children and Young Persons and their Families Agency, we find the same reticence to be a part of that complement. One of the several TV programs concerning this case was an excellent discussion on the early evening Holmes show. He had two people in the studio who were obviously in favour of the stand which the boys parents were taking in following the alternative method of treatment for their son. He also had a doctor in our Capital City of Wellington who he could switch into and bring on screen. It was even more obvious that he was totally anti-alternative and assured his viewers that Liam should be returned immediately to the hospital to be given more chemotherapy, even to the extent of making it quite clear that if this was not done, the boy would die.

At the end of the program, Paul Holmes asked the two in his studio if they were in favour of working with the medical people if this could be achieved, and they both made it quite clear that they would be happy to see this happen. Paul then switched the doctor in Wellington on to the screen and asked him if he would be prepared to work in conjunction with the alternative people who were now treating Liam. His answer to that question did not take very long to give to us. It consisted of just two letters. NO.

It is as if we have a river which people badly need to be able to cross. On one side you have a very keen group who have enough of the necessary facilities to build half of the bridge from their side to the centre of the river, and are very happy to do so, but on the other side another group are refusing to build their half, preferring to keep themselves to themselves. A little co-operation and a large helping of common sense would very soon solve the problem, but the two can never become one without those very necessary ingredients. Maybe you now have a better understanding of my reason for titling this chapter, "Bridging the Gap"

Before this is able to become a reality, it would seem to me that it will be necessary for science, as we know it to gain a greater understanding of energy. I have said before, but I want to say it again, there is nothing else in an endless universe but energy in its many forms and frequencies of vibration, and without this understanding it is not possible to be at one with anyone who uses energy to restore the damaged cells of an ailing body. Universal Energy, Love force, God force, whatever name you like to give it, it is the high frequency power of the universe which can restore those cells which become out of phase with the rest of the cells in the body. Bring them back into phase again by the use of this energy, and the body will once again be at ease instead of diseased.

For that is what disease is. Cells which for one reason or another have ceased to vibrate at the frequency at which they would normally keep the body in what we refer to as good health. A perfectly healthy body is simply one in which every living cell is vibrating at precisely its allotted rate, so therefore any variation in the frequency of vibration of any group of cells in that body will automatically cause some distress or discomfort to that body. If being unwell is as simple as having some cells in your body not vibrating at the correct frequency, then healing that body is also just as simple as restoring those cells to their normal vibratory rate. It should surely become very obvious then, that bringing them into unison with the rest of the cells would be more easily achieved by surrounding them with a measure of pure universal energy applied by the hands of a healer rather than attempting to do this by adding a chemical to the body in the form of a pill or a drug of some kind.

This energy being a totally natural part of all that is, can in no way have a deleterious effect on those cells. While the chemical may or may not have the desired effect on them there is every possibility that it may also create an imbalance in other cells. How often have we heard of a patient who has been prescribed a particular medicine for a problem in their body, and are then given something else to take to counteract some effect the first one has had on them.

While I was staying in Vermont in '98 my organiser for the trip presented me with a book which she thought I may find interesting. It was written by Nicole Lavoie, and is titled "Return to Harmony". I am sure Nicole will not mind if I quote a few lines here from her book just to show you how others are coming to the same conclusions about health as I have been bringing to you on the pages of this book. "We know that everything is made up of the same basic elements, and is connected to everything else. We are all one. Our bodies appear to be very solid, yet in the truth, they consist of atoms that are full of space. We are mostly space, with everything else vibrating at a certain frequency or rate. It is all vibration, and where every tiny part is doing its job and vibrating in harmony, we are healthy. Now imagine that a belief, a fear, an accident, lack of proper nutrition, or some other form of stress, caused us to lower our vibratory rate. Because everything is 'Vibration and Energy' this lowered vibratory rate caused part of our body to alter its vibration, then forget its role and stop functioning properly."

My word, haven't we seen that almost identical explanation somewhere before? I know they do say, "Great minds think alike", but I do not for one moment consider I have a great mind, only an OPEN one. And when scientists and medical people finally open their minds to this simple level of understanding, we will have reached the stage where the gap which presently stands between us will have been bridged, and together we will be able to work for the good of mankind. I look forward to that time with great anticipation, and vow to continue to do my utmost to attempt to bring it about sooner rather than later.

It is necessary for this to take place as soon as possible in order that those who, like our little girl with her six or seven fits a day, and so many others who continue to suffer only because their doctors have failed to find the source of their problem, will no longer find themselves in that position as the realisation of the importance of the vibratory rate of the cells of the body becomes fully accepted. Nicole also mentions the importance of developing ways to bridge what she refers to as the scientific and spiritual communities. Many people are joining together with the common goal of merging science and Spirit. The separation we used to think was so real is gradually proving to be only an illusion, an illusion that will soon fade into history.

`Near the beginning of this chapter I mentioned the phone call I received one evening from the organiser of a group where I had travelled to lecture and to teach about two weeks previously. She rang to tell me that a number of the students I had taught had gathered together to have their first practise, and to assure me that everything had gone off very well. But since that time I have now received a letter from her with some photos which she took at the public meeting we held there. I have produced one of these for you on Page 128. It was taken at a time when I was doing a demonstration of Magnetic Healing on a patient after the slides had been shown.

I would like you to take a good close look at this photo and note the expressions on the faces of what would have been about half of the number of people at that meeting. For many of these people this would have been the first time they had ever seen anyone being worked on by a healer in this way. I am sure they must have been thinking it was very different to anything they had ever seen in a doctor's surgery which most of them would normally visit if they were ill. But I do not think that you could say there was even one face there which would give you the impression that they were bored with the proceedings. I think you will agree that they all appear to be watching with great interest something which they had never experienced before.

In the short note which came with this photo, she mentioned that she was now healing on a regular basis about four days a week, and enjoying it more and more, and thanked me for having shown her the way. She also assured me that the "Energy Check" or "Aurameter" which she bought from me when I was there was terrific. She said it was like a teacher who was confirming for her that what she feels with her hand in the way of negative energy, really is precisely at that point. It is this degree of accuracy which confirms for a student that they really are on the right path, which makes this instrument so popular. I always feel good when I receive a letter from someone I have shown the way of healing, when that letter tells me that she is now actually carrying on with the practical work of using her newfound knowledge and ability to help those in need. Surely actions speak more loudly than words, and a portion of an article in a Theosophy magazine received a few days ago bears this out very well.

"In one of the Upanishads, is the story of an aspirant going to a great teacher and requesting him to enlightenment him on Brahman. The teacher asks him to tell him about his progress so far, and what he has learnt. In reply the aspirant gives a very elaborate account of all the Scripture that he has learnt. The teacher smiles and says, "These are merely words, but Brahman has to be experienced". Similarly, the chanting of mantras or recitation of hymns results in only a limited benefit. "Any approach, either on the path of knowledge or on the path of devotion must result in an experience beyond words, an experience which transcends the senses and the mind."

Yes my friend, words are cheap. They can flow with little effort from ones lips, but actions such as freely giving your time and your energy by reaching out your hands to one in need will surely show you that actions truly do speak more loudly than any words you could ever speak. When you begin to make the effort to seek the eternal truth, it is as if you are stirring the Universal Energy within yourself and placing your feet firmly on the next rung of the ladder of evolvement.

In some of my other books I have quoted from messages which had been channelled through from Spirit by a lovely lady I knew as "Illiana" and had the pleasure of staying with in the US in 1985. She had been producing a little magazine for some years under the name of "New Age Teachings". It consisted entirely of messages which she had channelled over a long period of time, and during my visit to her home I had the pleasure and privilege of sitting with her and listening to one of these messages tumbling from her lips as she sat in a trance state in front of a small group of interested seekers. This lady has now returned from whence those messages were coming through to her, and no doubt she will have joined some of those in Spirit who had been the source of many wonderful messages of wisdom over so many years. In memory of her and the wonderful work she did to help to bring Spiritual awareness and an upliftment of body mind and soul for so many throughout her life in the physical, I would like to copy here just one of the hundreds of messages which were recorded on tape then printed in her magazine.

"Suns of light, at this time we will explain to you the Cosmic scientific way in which Healing Energy operates to bring a sense of harmony and balance to those who 'tune in' to the correct vibrations. Divine energy is everywhere and acts as a strong magnet. It is made up of the positive vibrations of all the rays of light who have returned to the source. It is a pure Magnetic Force truly operating in the universe to aid struggling humanity to achieve a renewed state of harmony and balance.

For a few moments think about the physical magnet you are so familiar with. Observe how it attracts certain responsive objects. Now go a step further and think about other human beings who you know, and ponder how certain ones have a magnetic quality about them. Those who are materialists attract money and wealth. Those who are musical attract music energy to themselves, becoming fine musicians. Those who have violent magnetic qualities attract danger to their lives, and those who are Spiritually Magnetic attract light and are bestowed with Cosmic blessings and Spiritual beauty. The latter is Spiritual energy of the highest order, and it is this which we know as Cosmic Magnetic Energy. This is the energy you are to reach for. All true saints are forever filled with this energy and are the instruments through which this divine energy works and distributes itself to the energy starved beings reaching out in their consciousness for the revitalising rays to heal them.

Now to explain how energy does its work. When a human entity is either physically ill or emotionally disturbed, or is Spiritually starved, it means that through some error he or she has disconnected the life support system from the source. Once they consciously realise the need to be re-attached to divine energy, he or she will contact a Spiritual healing channel who will act as the intermediary to re-attach the life support system to the one who is ailing. You see, through conscious Spiritual direction the healing channel can visualise the golden stream of electrifying light energy as it beams forth directly from his or her being to the one who seeks the healing. You must understand that the magnetic divine force is attached to every entity. It is only disconnected when the entity disconnects himself or herself through ignorant acts which disturbs body, mind, soul function. Therefore to be re-attached again requires a positive effort on the entities part. He/she must have a strong belief in the principle of Cosmic Light, a strong and positive attitude, and strong and abiding patience. All of this, with the assistance of an illumined channel, will eventually bring the desired result.

It must be realised however, that in each case the magnetic force will reach out differently. And it is so important to remember that the openness of the entity has much to do with the speed that energy re-enters the total being. If one is doubtful or resistful then he or she is not a good magnet to attract the divine particles to himself. But one who is understanding of this divine magnetic law will be a well prepared instrument and very quickly there will begin the transformation desired which brings balance and harmony to the body-mind-soul being.

It is important also to speak to you about becoming a Spiritual Magnetic Force that can be a helpful instrument of light aiding others not yet fully attuned to this Magnetic Force. Once you fully comprehend the divine principle employed, you can fortify your own Magnetic Field. To do this you must mingle with bright suns who have already achieved a strong magnetic quality. Commune with them often, gathering from them divine ions which will strengthen your own magnetic field. If you are preparing to become a healing channel or a communication channel it is very important that you develop great divine magnetic strength. Then you will not only be a beneficent worker for light, but you will also be protected against the few who may enter your force field to drain your energy."

Through most of this book I have been bringing to you an understanding of healing as we see it from our physical level here on the earth plane, but the foregoing message which Illiana channelled a few years ago brings with it an overview of this work as it is seen from that other level of existence we refer to as the Spirit world. I am sure you will agree it contains many wise words and suggestions for anyone who is contemplating becoming a healer. And of course, as I would expect, it makes no secret of the fact that this is something which should not be treated lightly. You are setting out to become one with divine energy in order to be able to have the privilege of channelling it to those whose vibratory rate has fallen to a level which has brought about a condition which we call disease or discomfort of some kind in the body.

You cannot expect to be able to raise their vibration to a level which will eliminate the problem which they are suffering if you have not already made a supreme effort to bring your own vibratory rate up to a level which will allow you to pass the necessary degree of high frequency energy to your patient in order to achieve the desired result. You must begin with yourself. A strong flow of water will not flow through a rusty and leaking pipe, so do not expect an abundance of that divine magnetic healing energy which Illianas guide spoke of to flow freely through a channel which is only half-hearted about the work he or she is doing. You must raise your conscious awareness of your true soul-self within to new heights of acceptance. Doubts bring blockages, and total recognition of your oneness with all that is can remove them. That which you achieve, will be in direct proportion to the depth of your desire to serve.

How deep is your desire? Are you prepared to accept ridicule from those who think they know that what you are doing is impossible? Are you afraid you may lose a few friends because they consider you have become a little strange? These things and more can become reality when it becomes known that you think you can heal people, when as I have been told, you are not even a doctor. But remember, it is only those who have stubbornly refused to open their minds to anything which would appear to be outside the traditional boundaries of science who think this way. And do realise that this is their loss not yours. It is them who are refusing to climb the ladder of evolvement in this incarnation, and are not aware that if they remain that way throughout, then they must return in another body in a new incarnation at another time in order to learn the lessons which they have failed to experience in this one.

Do not waste the valuable time you have been allotted in this incarnation by frittering it away having what is commonly referred to as a good time. Get your priorities right. Realise why you have been given this time and what you are supposed to do with it. 'By their deeds ye shall know them' is a well known quote from the Bible, and I am sure there was a good reason for having it there. What have you done today to help someone in need? You may tell me you are not a healer so there was nothing you could do. But be aware that even a word of encouragement in the ear of someone who is feeling down for some reason can raise that ones vibration and help them to see the positive side of life instead of always concentrating on the negative. Let your light shine for all to see, and allow some of that light to rub off on all you meet or come in contact with. Once you have raised your consciousness to a level where you have that total recognition of your oneness with 'all that is', then you find there is no limit to the endless energy which is available for you to draw on and pass on to any who so desire it, whether their need is physical, mental or Spiritual.

Did I hear someone say, what do you mean when you say 'All that is'? How many words would you like me to use to explain that? How would just one do? God. Did he not say the kingdom of God is within you? How then can there be any barriers between you and the 'all that is' if you are a part of it? Leave the limitations behind you and step into that higher frequency level of existence which knows no bounds. A level where "Miracles" become the norm, and the doubts and fears which have held you in their grasp for so long become a thing of the past.

I had thought that maybe I had already quoted from more than enough letters in this book, but one which arrived in the mail this morning appears to be crying out for me to quote just a few lines from it in view of what I have just been saying about those doubts and fears which stifle your advancement. "Dear Mr Lambert, I am reading your book "Magnetic Healing and Other Realities", and can hardly wait to finish it so I can start again. I got it from our library last week. I find the message so timely and so simple. I am so glad I found it. It is a bit tatty so it must have been well read. I have been a 'Christian' for over 30 years and really made no progress until very recently. I don't even like to call myself that any more. What a far cry from truth and reality is the system out there."

Oh dear! Did I step on somebody's toes there. Well I am sorry, but I was only passing on to you what are obviously the very strong feelings of a lady who would appear to be rejoicing over the fact that after 30 years of being chained to dogmatic beliefs which she was expected to totally embrace whether she could find any proof that they had any basis in truth or not, has finally broken the chains and can now begin to use that wonderful thing her creator gave her to think with. Now she can raise her conscious awareness of her true soul-self within and recognise her oneness with that which I previously referred to as the 'All that is'.

Many times over the years a patient has entered my healing room and asked me if I am a Christian. There is only one answer you can give to anyone who comes up with that question. You were afraid I was going to say, "no" weren't you. But that is not the answer I give them at all. My reply to that question is to ask them to sit down and define for me, a Christian. Strange to say, in many cases I find the one who asked the question is now at a total loss for words. It seems to be that as long as I assure them I am a Christian, then that is fine, and they are quite happy to step onto the couch and have me work on them. But ask them to define one, and that becomes a very different story. I have long since realised that people have very different ideas about what constitutes a Christian. Some think that if you go to church on Sunday, then you must be a good Christian, but I have not always found that to be true by any means. A business man who goes to church on Sunday because it makes him look like a good honest man to deal with, may well be just the one who is waiting to rob you on some deal on Monday.

Perhaps if we were to return to that little quote I made from the Bible a short time ago we may well be looking at something more like the truth. I am not suggesting there are no genuine honest people in a church by any means, but what I am saying is that just because someone goes to church or belongs to a particular religion, that does not necessarily make him a good Christian. If I was ever asked to consider whether a particular person was what we may think of as being a good Christian, then I would not just want to look at what they did with their Sundays, but would want to take note of that ones thoughts, words and actions towards their fellow beings for every day of the week. Yes, it has been well said, 'By their deeds ye shall know them'.

It was my intention to bring this book to a close with the preceding thoughts, but a short item which was a part of the Holmes show on our TV a couple of nights ago cries out for inclusion. Perhaps it would have been more appropriate for it to have been included in chapter three, 'Doors Begin to Open'. But I am sure in a book titled 'Healers Unlimited' it will not be out of place here and will be a fitting end for a book which is mainly designed to bring to the notice of its readers just how quickly the unorthodox or alternative is gaining recognition as a viable complement to the orthodox.

We were taken into the large hospital in Wellington city, New Zealand's Capital, where we were treated to the scene of a nurse laying her hands on one of the patients to remove pain and discomfort from his body. Nurse Bridget Hayden had been to Colorado and learnt a method of healing known as 'Healing Touch'. She explained that if one of your family is having a problem with their health it is quite common for many people to simply place a hand on that one in an attempt to help to relieve the pain, and that is fine. But here we were seeing something which had gone well beyond that. Here was one who had been placing her hands on a body, and consciously applying the energy to that body. That in itself is good to see being shown on any TV program, but when it is being carried out in one of our countries largest hospitals with the blessing of the medical staff, then that becomes a very different story.

We were informed that the doctors there were embracing the treatment, and that the patients could not get enough of it. One cancer patient who was interviewed assured us he had physical improvement, and we were told that what was happening here was opening a new age of health care, not in a health centre, but in Wellington hospital. At first nurse Hayden was labelled the 'Airy-fairy' nurse, but now she has a growing following and has trained seventy other nurses to meet the demand. We were shown a man who had a leg amputated at the knee. His mother told us she had placed her hands where the leg was missing and suddenly felt a stabbing energy pulsating into the palm. She felt she had caught her sons phantom pain, and this happened to be borne out by the fact that her son has not needed to take any pain killers since that time. A lady with cancer said she could feel the balance coming back into her life, and the treatment had been deeply relaxing.

A doctor who spoke to us concerning what was taking place here said that traditional medicine was backing the alternative approach. While he did not feel that it was actually healing the patients, he pointed out that it was certainly having a positive effect on the patients well being, and helping them cope with complex cancer therapy. Wellington hospital says it hopes other hospitals will follow its lead. The program concluded with the following statement. "The success of medical procedure is measured by results, and so far the results of Healing Touch are becoming hard to ignore".

No doubt you can see why this piece of information should have been in the chapter which was devoted to informing you how doors were beginning to open, but as they say, better late than never. While I enjoyed watching the program and making sure that I was recording it on video tape so that I would have the exact words to copy from, I was also struck by what was for me, the irony of its contents. I realise you may well be wondering why, after so many years of attempting to bring the truth of healing to as many people as possible, I should find a program such as this to be in any way, ironic.

I guess it was just the fact that as I watched it and saw doctors in one of our largest hospitals embracing this new approach to bringing health to their patients, it was difficult not to look back and remember the two occasions on which my work as a healer had been shown on our TV. In 1974 when I had been instrumental in bringing to the screen the healing work which the Psychic Surgeons were doing in Manila and my time spent working with them, plus the 1998 fiasco with our little Maori girl and her epileptic fits, were both an orchestrated attempt to portray any form of healing as being of little or no use to the viewers. Yet suddenly, here we were watching a program which was going to every bit as much trouble to prove to the viewers that healing with the hands really does work.

After being chased away on so many occasions by doctors, both in hospitals and out, it was hard to believe that I really was watching doctors in a hospital openly admitting that this work was having a positive effect on the patients well-being, and stating that they hoped other hospitals would follow their lead. How could such opposing views have suddenly surfaced for all to see and hear? One conclusion I did come to took me back to a statement I have made elsewhere. I have said many times that there is no point in saying something unless you are somebody, because nobody takes any notice. What doctor would want to 'waste their time' as our Starship Hospital doctor had put it, talking to someone who was 'not even a doctor'. Especially someone who had twenty or more years running his own painting and paperhanging business before claiming he had discovered that he could heal people with his hands simply by 'Pulling and drawing away aches and diverse impurities' precisely as the great Hippocrates was doing so many years ago.

But it soon became very obvious to me that to be a trained nurse rather than a painter was enough to give the whole thing that little bit of extra authenticity. Enough for the medical people to consider at least looking at it to see whether there really was anything to be gained by embracing something which at first sight must have appeared to be well outside the traditional boundaries of science. Having to admit their patients were showing positive effects from the healing must have been the icing on the cake for the nurses who were being used as channels for the healing energy. One more reason for the doctors being able to accept what was taking place in their hospital stood out very strongly for me, and it is this particular aspect which I want to say a few words about before I lay down my pen.

You may have noticed that this type of healing is called "Healing Touch', and of course it is not something which is new to me, having heard of others being trained in this way before. There are many ways of using the Love Force energy to heal the sick. I have already mentioned the psychic surgeons in the Philippines who use the energy to open the body and physically remove dross from it such as a cancer growth. But on my bookshelf you would find quite a collection of books which describe the different ways of using this energy to bring new health to ailing bodies. One of these is titled "Therapeutic Touch" by Dr Dolores Kreiger, and another by Mary Coddington is called "In Search of the Healing Energy". This one has the following statement written on the cover. " Take a look into the future when the proper manipulation of the healing energy will bring about a revolution in medicine." All of these and many others written by authors living in different areas in the world recognise the basic fact that there is energy in its many forms and frequencies throughout an endless universe, waiting for us to recognise it, accept it, and use it for the good of mankind.

But looking along the shelf my eye falls on one which is of particular interest to me at this time, because the name on the front of this one simply says, "Healing Touch". 'A resource for health care professionals', by Dorothea Hover-Kramer. This of course, is exactly what we saw our nurse using on our TV program. This book contains some very good quotes such as the following. "If all matter is really energy, as Einstein insists, then we must see the human body as a dynamic interactive energy system and develop ways to work with the energy for healing." Another shorter but just as much to the point statement says, "Energy is the real substance of matter and form". All of these books and many more have very much in common, and they all explain how the healing energy can be applied to an ailing body to minimise the pain and suffering, and, as the Wellington doctor put it, have a positive effect on the patients well-being.

But in most cases this appears to be where they draw the line and do not appear to be aware that so much more can be achieved if only the healer will believe and know that the only limits to the healing work, are the ones we place there with our own ignorance of the potential which lies waiting for us to recognise it and to use it. Perhaps I was fortunate in spending at least eight weeks during '74 and '75 working with the Psychic Surgeons in Manila. At that time I had only done a small amount of healing, but that experience taught me that I should never place limits on what we can do if we can gain a deep enough understanding of the limitless achievements which are possible when we learn how to become one with the ever present energy.

I am sure it was those weeks of helping with hundreds of operations. Watching Romy Bugarin or one of the other healers open a body and remove anything from a clot to a cancer growth before asking me to run the palm of my hand over the opening and watch it close, which created within me that extra level of acceptance which allowed me to develop what I have called Magnetic Healing. It helped to develop within me the understanding that instead of just touching the body in many places and allowing the energy to flow into it to bring balance and harmony to the body, the hand could be moved along through the energy field surrounding it, and that it would only stop moving when it reached the area immediately above the SOURCE of the problem. I came to realise this was the only place where any great amount of time and energy needed to be used. And perhaps even more importantly I learnt that while I may not have the ability to open the body and physically remove the unwanted dross from a body, I could use this energy to speed up the vibratory rate of the unwanted atoms and draw them up through a so-called solid body in the form of, as our six year old Maori girl put it, "a lump of black meat" and throw it away in the corner of the room.

Strange though it may seem it is actually this recognition of what can be done when we understand something about energy which has brought about my "Downfall". I had better explain that one carefully because you are probably thinking something like, 'I didn't know he had fallen down'. By 'downfall', I simply mean my inability to break through the barriers of orthodox medical practise to any great extent. You see, while doctors such as those in Wellington Hospital may be willing to accept that a nurse with a deep desire to help an ailing patient to feel better by placing their hands on them and allowing some mysterious energy flow through to bring about a positive effect on the patients well being, to suggest that something like an ulcer or a cancer growth can actually be removed as mentioned above is much too large a step for one trained in orthodox medical practise to ever consider taking.

Perhaps you could say this is where this word 'irony' comes in again. If I had approached medical people some years ago and told them I could help to relieve the pain in their patients and help them to heal more quickly after an operation, then perhaps I would have been able to receive an acceptance of that. What I did not realise was the fact that I was attempting to go too far too fast. But now that doctors are prepared to accept that this energy does exist, and that it can be beneficial in removing pain and discomfort from their patients, then perhaps the next step will be for them to begin looking at the endless possibilities which already lie within the framework of magnetic Healing.

It is of course, one of those which has to pass through those three phases. We have almost passed through the years of being scoffed at, and now as we slowly but surely move into the time of being tolerated, I look forward with great anticipation to that joyous time when it will be accepted as an obvious truth. Be sure, you do your part in helping to bring that into reality.

Appendix to Magnetic Healers

The following is a short list of some of Colin's students who are now practising Magnetic Healing. If you have a problem with your health, give one near you a ring, it could be the most rewarding call you have ever made.

NEW ZEALAND - North Island

Whangarei

John & Margaret Walton, 3/2 Elizabeth Street	09 437 1966

Auckland

Jacqui Oliver, 16 Blenheim Street, Glenfield	09 480 7733
Mark Tyrrell, Onehunga	09 636 3174
Lorraine Allen, Parnell	09 302 2252
Steve Gailey, 47 Malvern Road, Mt Albert	09 849 2761
David & Juanita Brown, 29 Rena Place, West Harbour, Waitakere City	09 416 7857

Tauranga

Craig Lankshear	07 578 1049

Opotiki

Diane Collins, 68 Grant Road	07 315 7019 A/H07 315 6810
Kris Hillier, 5/107 Richard Street	07 315 6974
Mininui Peni, Tirohanga Beach, SH 35	07 315 6045
John Schiavi	025 247 2765
Cherry Wood, 92 Grant Road	07 315 5842
Lynda Farnworth, PO Box 567, Waioweka Gorge	025 493 415
Chris Buckland, Tutaetoka Road	07 315 6153

Pirongia

Des Barr, Boffin Street	07 871 9976

Te Awamutu

David Holland, 395 Elizabeth Street	07 871 3414

Te Kuiti

Carolyn Dutton, "Carolyns" 233 Rora Street	07 878 7030

Stratford

Valerie Burton, 26 Olivia Street	06 765 6833

Wairoa

Lorraine Horsfield, 2 Kauri Street	06 838 7826

Hastings

Margaret Turner, 1230 Norfolk Crescent	06 876 9369

Palmerston North

Kathy Moore, Palmerston North Healing	06 354 9317
Centre Director and Co-ordinator	
"Magnetic Healers Unlimited"	021 217 3732
Christine Dawson	06 356 4075
Sean Hogue, Healer@xtra.co.nz	06 357 6942
Pamela Howell, PHOWELL@xtra.co.nz	06 358 9354

Wanganui

Fiona Britton, Taylor Road, Tayforth RD 4	06 347 2388 021 445 687
Brenda Grundy, 12 Hurworth Place	06 345 6774

New Plymouth

Zeta Peters, 189b Parkland Ave Bell Block	06 755 1434 025 477 760
Les Davidson	06 753 9800

Upper Hutt

Bruce Goodall, 56 Whakatiki Street	04 528 7743

NEW ZEALAND - South Island

Jill Hollis, Pakawau, RD 1Golden Bay	03 524 8401
Peter Gillies, Takaka	025 247 3609
Graham Fraser, Westhaven Inlet, Golden Bay	025 252 1555
Lou Moser, Bainham RD 1	03 524 8577

Blehheim

Zeta Maxted	03 578 5906

North Otago

Val Kerry, 37 Derby Street, Hampden	021 517 136

Christchurch

Dave & Eva Mason, 13 Hays Rise, Governors Bay	03 329 9727

Dunedin

George Mawdsley	03 474 9099 025 223 4828

South Canterbury

Reg Simpson, 66 Cox Street, Geraldine	03 693 9885

AUSTRALIA

Perth, Western Australia

Carol Duffield, 9 Hotchin Way, Kardinja 6163	89 314 2030

Brisbane, Queensland

John Darling, PO Box 3117, Newstead 4006 Email - jgdarl@bit.net.au	07 3852 3162 fax 07 385 3262 Mobile 041 878 8300
Phil Bennet, 1/11 Bryant Street, Ashgrove 4060	Mobile 041 447 8448
Ron & Diane Yates, 20 Lincoln Court, Tullamore Downs, Beaudesert 4285	07 5541 4988

Nowra, New South Wales

Helen & Barry Turner, 7 Burrandool Avenue
North Nowra, NSW 2541 — 02 4422 1451

UNITED STATES

Vermont

Lisa Maxurkewich, PO Box 1212, Stowe Vermont 05672 — 802 253 9884

Bernice Kelman, 12 Kelly Road, Underhill Vermont 05489

John H Euber, PO Box 429, Hinesburg, Vermont 05461

Annie DiSpirito, Burlington, Vermont 05401

Arizona

Lavell Evans, PO Box 871, Bisbee 85603

New Mexico

Rod & Amy Sorrell, 204 West Riverside
Truth or Consequences NM 87901 — 800 982 0732

CANADA

Miss Jody Cavanaugh
West Bay Marina, 453 Head Street,
Victoria BC V9 A 531 — 1 250 381 1663, Mobile: 250 885 7084

Mrs Clare Dick, 4641 Fairlawn,
Burnaby BC V5C 3R5 — 1 604 299 0612

Mrs Zoe Klassen
604 Berry Street, Coquitlam BC V3J 5T6 — 1 604 936 9093, Mobile: 1 604 862 2071

Mrs Marilyn Parkin
Apartment 115, 5374 203rd Street
Langley BC V3A 7J8 — 1 604 530 7954, Fax: 1 604 530 7938